Principles of
Social Research

Edited by Judith Green and John Browne

Open University Press

Open University Press
McGraw-Hill Education
McGraw-Hill House
Shoppenhangers Road
Maidenhead
Berkshire
England
SL6 2QL

email: enquiries@openup.co.uk
world wide web: www.openup.co.uk

and Two Penn Plaza, New York, NY 10121-2289, USA

First published 2005
Reprinted 2006

A catalogue record of this book is available from the British Library

ISBN–10: 0 335 21835 0
ISBN–13: 978 0 335 21835 6

Library of Congress Cataloguing-in-Publication Data
CIP data applied for

Typeset by RefineCatch Ltd, Bungay, Suffolk
Printed in the UK by Bell and Bain

Contents

Acknowledgements

Open University Press and the London School of Hygiene and Tropical Medicine have made every effort to obtain permission from copyright holders to reproduce material in this book and to acknowledge these sources correctly. Any omissions brought to our attention will be remedied in future editions.

We would like to express our grateful thanks to the following copyright holders for granting permission to reproduce material in this book.

page 64   Coreil J, 'Group Interview Methods in Community Health Research,' Medical Anthropology, 16: 193 210 (1995). © Taylor & Francis Ltd. Journals website: http:/www.tandf.co.uk/journals

Overview of the book

Introduction

The problems facing public health are increasingly those of human behaviour. At an individual level there are problems of developing more effective models of health promotion to encourage healthier lifestyles; at the level of society there are problems of understanding the effects of social change on health, or what the barriers are to effective policy implementation. Increasingly, public health practitioners and managers are turning to social research to help understand human behaviour.

This book introduces some of the principles of social research as applied to public health. It is aimed at those with some understanding of health and health care, but little exposure to social research. It does not, therefore, aim to provide readers with all the skills that they would need to carry out a social research study; rather, it aims to develop their understanding of the key principles involved.

The contribution of social science to public health has not just been to introduce a 'tool box' of research techniques such as focus groups or survey designs. It has also brought a set of disciplinary perspectives that are in many ways different from those of biomedicine. This book introduces some of the social science disciplines that have turned their attention to health and health care. The main areas drawn on here are medical sociology (which has informed much qualitative research in health and health services research, particularly in high income countries) and psychology (which has made a major contribution in particular to more quantitative methods). The theoretical contributions of these disciplines are not discussed in this book. We focus primarily on using particular qualitative and quantitative methods.

Why study the principles of social research?

Not everyone has to (or wants to!) carry out social research, but most people in public health will at some point have to read the findings of others and assess how useful they are for their own practice. They may also need to commission social research, or collaborate with researchers from the disciplines introduced here. After studying this book, readers will develop their understanding of how to assess social research, by grasping such issues as the choice of appropriate design and the strengths and weaknesses of particular data collection methods. Readers will also develop their understanding of the various perspectives from which social scientists approach research, aiding their ability to contribute to multidisciplinary public health practice.

Structure of the book

This book follows the conceptual outline of the Principles of Social Research unit at the London School of Hygiene & Tropical Medicine. It is based on the materials presented in the lectures and seminars of the taught course, which have been adapted for distance learning.

There are four sections in this book, containing 16 chapters. Each chapter includes:

- an overview
- a list of learning objectives
- a list of key terms
- a range of activities
- feedback on the activities
- a summary.

The following description of the section and chapter contents will give you an idea of what you will be studying.

Social science and research

In the first section we introduce the social sciences, the principles of research design and the debate about what 'science' might mean in this context. The chapters in this section aim to orientate the reader to the general problems faced in turning a topic of interest into a question that can be answered through research, and then designing a particular project that can answer it.

Qualitative methods

This section and the next are about 'methods' and are concerned with different kinds of research design and methods of collecting data. For convenience we have divided them into qualitative methods and quantitative methods, although we recognize that, in practice, this division may not be a very convincing one. The chapters in this section are not an exhaustive discussion of methods but aim to introduce the most common data collection methods used in qualitative research in health, including interviews, focus groups and participant observation. We include an introduction to qualitative analysis to aid understanding of qualitative research outputs.

Quantitative methods

As with the preceding section, the chapters in this section are not an exhaustive discussion of methods but aim to introduce the most common data collection methods used in quantitative research in health, including questionnaires and surveys. We have not covered statistical analysis: many public health practitioners are more familiar with the principles of quantitative analysis and discussion of statistical methods is outside the scope of this text.

Anthropology and history

Two other disciplines, medical anthropology and the history of medicine, have also had a long tradition of contribution to and collaboration with public health. Their contribution has been primarily that of offering a new perspective on issues in public health, and we have therefore introduced these disciplines in separate chapters in the final section. The chapters on medical anthropology and history are, therefore, orientated towards illustrating the approaches of anthropology and history as well as the particular research techniques used. Finally, recognizing that much public health research uses a range of methods, often drawn from more than one discipline, we discuss some of the issues raised by integrating some of the methods and disciplines covered in the book within the same project.

Acknowledgements

The authors acknowledge the contribution of Clive Seale, Professor of Sociology at Brunel University, for detailed comments and advice, and Deirdre Byrne (series manager) for help and support.

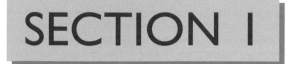

SECTION I

Introduction

1 Introduction to social research

Judith Green and John Browne

Overview

For many people trained as health professionals or managers, the terms and concepts used by social scientists are unfamiliar and difficult to apply to the 'real life' practical problems that they need to address in their working lives. The chapters in this first section introduce you to some of the language used by social scientists, and provide an opportunity to reflect on how social research methods could be used to address issues raised by public health practice. These chapters introduce the social sciences, the concept of scientific research and research design. They will explore how the methods of social scientists can be used to study health and health behaviour. The aims of the section are to provide the skills needed to identify when social research methods can contribute to our understanding of health and health care systems, to develop research questions and to identify appropriate research designs for answering them.

This chapter introduces the social science disciplines that will be discussed in this book and outlines how they can contribute to research in public health.

Learning objectives

After studying this chapter you will be better able to:

- **identify how social science research methods can contribute to our understanding of public health and health management problems**
- **distinguish between qualitative and quantitative research methods**

Key terms

Method A set of strategies for asking useful questions, designing a study, collecting data and analysing data.

Methodology The study of the principles of investigation, including the philosophical foundations of choice of methods.

Qualitative Pertaining to the nature of phenomena: how they are classified.

Quantitative Pertaining to the measurement of phenomena.

What is social science?

By 'social research methods' we mean methods developed within the social sciences. Social science is a general term for the study of aspects of human behaviour. It includes many disciplines. Those you will come across in this book are:

- sociology
- anthropology
- psychology
- history.

These disciplines have different interests, theoretical approaches, origins and favoured methods. However, they share a rigorous and systematic approach to research, and all have contributed to our understanding of health, health behaviour and health care. Some of the areas of health care that have interested social scientists include:

- assessing local needs for health care
- understanding the factors that influence people's decision to seek health care
- understanding why patients do or don't adhere to treatment regimes
- evaluating the health and quality of life of patients after treatment
- exploring how the behaviour of health care workers can impact on the implementation of policy.

In this book, you will explore how social research methods can be used to address issues that are relevant to your work in the health sector. As a health professional or manager you may not need to carry out your own research. But, in making decisions about health care needs, how to prioritize them and how your practice and services can meet them you will almost certainly have to evaluate the research findings of others and perhaps commission original research of your own. The first aim of this book is to provide you with some skills in identifying when a 'problem' is one that can be addressed by social science methods.

People's health status, health behaviour, and how they utilize health services (their health-seeking behaviour) are influenced by a complex range of factors, including inherited biological characteristics, lifestyle, social circumstances and economic factors. Understanding how health care systems can meet health care needs in an efficient, effective and acceptable way relies on an understanding of how these factors affect both health, and an individual's use of health services. The first activity asks you to reflect on where social sciences might fit into the range of possible explanations for health and health behaviour.

Activity 1.1

The following could be identified as possible causes for differences in rates of heart disease between different groups in the population. Which ones do you think are appropriate subjects for social scientists to study:

a) genetic factors
b) stress
c) lifestyle factors (such as rates of smoking and exercise)

d) luck
e) economic circumstances
f) access to health services?

↻ Feedback

Those that are related to human behaviour are (b), (c), (e) and (f). However, social scientists are also interested in people's attitudes to, for example, luck, and in issues such as how information about genetic risk is communicated to patients. Whether or not a topic is appropriate for social science methods depends more on the kind of question asked than on the area of interest.

Research methods

Having identified that an issue is one that is relevant to the social sciences, the next task is to decide what kind of research method is appropriate. A research method is a particular strategy for answering a research question. It includes:

- The formulation of a research question. This is discussed in Chapter 3.
- General design of the study (for instance, the type of people we select for inclusion in our study; the method we use to recruit these people; how many people we need in the study; whether these people will be randomly allocated to one treatment or another; whether we contact study participants on a number of occasions or just once). Chapter 4 discusses some of these issues of research design.
- Development of tools to gather data (such as a questionnaire for use in a survey, or a list of prompts to use in an interview).

Sociology, anthropology, history and psychology use a range of research methods and some methods are associated more with particular disciplines than others. Table 1.1 lists some examples of the kinds of general questions each discipline asks about health care, and the methods often (although not exclusively, and not always) used to collect data. There is considerable overlap in the approaches of the different social science disciplines, and in practice public health research programmes often draw on more than one discipline.

The choice of a method is influenced, although not dictated, by the aim of research – by what the researcher is trying to find out. However, there are other factors that influence the choice of method used, which come from the fundamental beliefs of the researcher about what knowledge is and how it can be known. In Chapter 2 you will find out more about different orientations towards knowledge and how they inform methods. This general study of methods is called *methodology*.

Much health research in practice uses a variety of disciplines or methods to address different aspects of the same problem, and as you work through this book it will become apparent that a multidisciplinary approach is often the most appropriate way to carry out research on many public health problems. There are so many influences on health and health behaviour that, to gain a full understanding,

Table 1.1 Social science disciplines and the study of health care

Discipline	Examples of research interests	Typical data collection methods used
Sociology	What impact do social factors have on health?	Face-to-face surveys.
	How do health professionals understand policy change?	In-depth interviews.
Anthropology	How does culture affect health behaviour?	Observation of 'natural' behaviour, either as participant or outsider.
	How do people conceptualize 'health'?	
History	How have health policies changed over time?	Analysis of historical documents.
	How have people in other times understood health?	Oral history.
Psychology	How do patients' attitudes affect their health behaviour?	Questionnaires (for attitudes)/analysis of 'routine' data (e.g. GP attendance) for behaviour.
	How do health interventions impact on psychological outcomes such as depression?	Interviews or Questionnaires.

an explanation is needed on a number of levels. In the example in Activity 1.1, the possible influences on heart disease are of course related – the amount of stress people experience may be influenced by their economic position, and their access to health services may be influenced by social factors such as income or gender. However, it is often impossible to study all these factors within the same study design. An important task in any kind of research is to identify a research question from the complex web of factors that impact on the issue of interest.

What is a research question?

As a health professional or manager, you may be faced with a variety of practice and policy problems. Carrying out research is not always an appropriate response. The next activity is designed to prompt you to think about when it might be appropriate to consider using research. This could involve:

- thinking about whether it is possible to carry out research on the question
- searching for research done by others that is relevant to your experience
- carrying out your own study
- commissioning a larger project from an experienced researcher.

Activity 1.2

Think about a problem you currently face in your workplace, or one you have faced recently. Did you consider either carrying out or commissioning your own research to help make a decision about what to do? Jot down the main reasons why you answered 'yes' or 'no'.

Feedback

If you answered 'no', some of the reasons might be:

- the solution was already well known but difficult to implement
- resource constraints
- a solution was needed quickly and there was no time to wait for research results
- there were no resources (such as skills, library facilities or personnel) to carry out research
- it was hard to think of an appropriate study design to answer the question

If you answered 'yes', some of the reasons might be:

- there was uncertainty about the best solution
- there were conflicting accounts of what the solution or even 'the problem' was
- carrying out research provided more time to develop an acceptable solution
- the research was perceived as relatively easy to perform (for example, it may have been possible to use data that had already been collected for other purposes)

Research is perhaps most appropriately carried out when there is uncertainty: when we recognize that we need to know more about a problem in order to solve it, or when we have identified a gap in our knowledge. In practice, however, there may be many other motivations for doing research, such as the furtherance of career aims, the furtherance of a political agenda, or for an agency to 'be seen to be doing something' about an intractable problem. Social research is relevant when the 'problem' relates to aspects of human attitudes or behaviour, either of individuals or of groups in society. As the effectiveness, efficiency and acceptability of health care systems are influenced by human behaviour and attitude at many levels, social research methods are often relevant.

Activity 1.3

In this activity you are asked to consider the problems faced by the manager of an accident and emergency department based at a busy urban hospital. First read the case scenario in the paragraph below.

Scenario

The accident and emergency department treats 70,000 new cases a year, and staff feel that the majority of these patients do not need hospitals to provide their treatment. These patients attend with minor illnesses or injuries that do not require emergency treatment and their needs could have been met in local primary care facilities. However, junior doctors tend to investigate and treat patients with minor problems intensively, and the department was overspent last year. The department has had some very bad publicity recently as local newspapers have reported that patients often wait up to 24 hours on trolleys before being found a bed and there have been high-profile cases of patient dissatisfaction with treatment received. Waits for treatment are very long, contributing to an often hostile environment in the waiting room. Nurse turnover is high and it has been difficult to recruit good staff. The management team meets tomorrow to discuss whether there is any research that could usefully address these problems.

Now think about what the areas of uncertainty are here for the manager and how they relate to human behaviour. Which questions would you suggest the team addresses? Consider investigating both the need for hospital care, and patient and staff attitudes. Jot down those that you think could be addressed through research.

Feedback

Compare your notes with the possibilities outlined below.

From the manager's perspective, there are a number of questions which could be researched.

Here are some of them.

On the need for hospital care:

a) Which patients can be safely treated at the primary care level?
b) How many of our patients are attending 'inappropriately'?
c) When is primary care unavailable, leaving patients having to go to hospital for treatment?
d) How could the primary care level cope with the influx of new patients?

On patient attitudes and behaviour:

e) Why do patients choose to attend the hospital for treatment?
f) What are the sources of patient dissatisfaction with current hospital care, and primary care?

On staff attitudes and behaviour:

g) Why do junior doctors treat patients with minor problems 'intensively', rather than treating more appropriately or referring back to primary care?
h) Why do nurses feel dissatisfied with working here?
i) What are the barriers to nurse recruitment?
j) What would improve staff morale?

You may have identified other questions, perhaps economic ones about how to reduce costs. Others might be about 'public relations', such as how to improve the public's perception of your hospital. Look at your list to check that your questions are about health care need and human behaviour, and that they address areas of uncertainty that could be clarified through research. Other questions raised by this scenario are also of interest to social scientists. These include examining the role of the media in presenting and contributing to the public 'image' of an institution, or investigating why patients and professionals appear to have different ideas about where to go for appropriate treatment for minor health care problems.

Quantitative or qualitative methods?

The questions listed in Activity 1.3 are diverse, and a range of methods would be needed to address them. One way of dividing them up is to separate them into questions that are best addressed by qualitative or quantitative methods.

Quantitative methods are best used for questions that relate to 'quantities': they are about counting or measuring events or phenomena (such as questions that start 'when?' 'which?' 'how many?' or 'how much?').

Qualitative methods are best used for questions that relate to the 'quality' of or variations in experience, or the meaning of experience for different people, such as questions starting with 'why?' or 'what?' Qualitative methods are primarily used to classify events or phenomena, such as the nature of patient dissatisfaction, or barriers to nurse recruitment.

 Activity 1.4

Which of the questions listed in the feedback for Activity 1.3 would be best addressed by quantitative methods and which by qualitative methods?

Feedback

Questions (a), (b) and (c) would be best addressed by quantitative methods (they are about measurement) and the rest by qualitative methods (they are about identifying a range of attitudes, developing strategies, or exploring the meaning of events).

Section 2 will introduce some of the qualitative methods used in the social sciences, and Section 3 will introduce quantitative methods. Qualitative research is more likely to use methods such as observation or in-depth interviewing, which produce words as data, whereas quantitative researchers are more likely to use face-to-face surveys or self-completed questionnaires, which produce numbers as data. However, the contrast between the two kinds of data collection methods should not be exaggerated and many researchers use both qualitative and quantitative techniques within a single research project. History, which is explored in Section 4, uses both qualitative and quantitative methods depending on the research question. In addition, you should be aware that researchers sometimes perform a quantitative analysis of data produced through qualitative techniques, for instance in counting the different themes that emerge in interviews or focus groups.

As you read the scenario in Activity 1.3, you may have drawn on your own experience of management or working in similar departments to think of some explanations and possible solutions for the accident and emergency department manager's problems. What can social research add to this kind of professional experience? Unlike personal experience, 'common sense' or anecdote, research seeks systematically to collect and analyse data, and has a commitment to examining 'counter-explanations', or alternative interpretations. This approach is sometimes characterized as 'scientific'. In the next chapter, you will examine what 'science' means, and why social research methodology is described as 'scientific', even though the research subject of interest is individual people or groups of people.

Summary

There are many social influences on health, health behaviour and the organization of health services. Social science can contribute to investigating these influences through research in disciplines such as sociology, anthropology, psychology and history. Social research addresses both qualitative questions, which explore the meaning of events and phenomena (how they are classified) and quantitative questions that address measurement (when, which, how often, or how much).

Further reading

Campbell O, Cleland J, Collumbien M and Southwick K (1999) *Social Science Methods for Research on Reproductive Health*. Geneva: WHO.

An excellent and practical introduction to designing and conducting social research in the field of reproductive health, with examples drawn widely from health care systems around the world.

Bowling A (1997) *Research Methods for Health: Investigating Health and Health Services*. Buckingham: Open University Press.

This is a comprehensive introduction to the range of methods used in health and health services research, including demography, epidemiology and economic approaches as well as other social science methods. It is particularly good on the more quantitative approaches.

2 | Science and social science
Judith Green and John Browne

Overview

In this chapter you will learn about some basic concepts in the philosophy of science – what science is, what makes a discipline 'scientific' and how knowledge becomes legitimate. Many students find these ideas difficult if they have had no previous contact with social sciences or other humanities, and have difficulty seeing why they are relevant to the study of research methods. However, some understanding of theories of how knowledge is produced and of the different principles underlying various approaches in the social sciences is essential for understanding the different aims of research, and how to judge the worth of research findings appropriately. If you find this chapter difficult at this point, or cannot see how it is relevant, don't worry, but try returning to it when you have finished the rest of the book. Some students find these ideas easier to think about when they can relate them to some substantive knowledge of health research studies.

Learning objectives

When you have completed this chapter, you will be better able to:

- **appreciate the social context of science**
- **identify different methodological approaches within the social sciences**

Key terms

Hypothesis A provisional explanation for the phenomena under study.

Positivism A philosophy of science which assumes that reality is stable and can be researched by measuring observable indicators.

Relativism An alternative to positivism, which assumes that reality can change depending on who is observing it and from where.

What is science?

✏ Activity 2.1

What does 'science' mean to you? What kinds of research would you describe as 'scientific'?

↻ Feedback

Science means different things to different people but for many the word has connotations of laboratories, experiments and people in white coats. Scientific research is often associated predominately with the 'natural' sciences such as biology, chemistry or physics, and is seen as an enterprise that generates objective knowledge about the world.

Research in the natural sciences is often perceived to be more 'objective' than that in the social sciences because scientists appear to agree on how to classify natural phenomena and how to study them. In the social sciences, by contrast, there is (as we have seen already) a range of approaches and methods, and findings can seem more 'subjective' in that their interpretation may depend on the approach taken by the attitudes of the researcher. In most contemporary societies, in most fields of endeavour (and certainly in medicine and health care), scientific knowledge has a status and legitimacy not afforded to other sources of knowledge: it is seen as more valid and credible than knowledge derived from non-scientific sources (such as personal experience, religious texts, or the wisdom of elders).

So what characterizes the 'scientific method' that produces this kind of legitimate knowledge about the world? Philosophers of science have disagreed on what makes science 'scientific' but many accounts focus on a number of features that are often seen to apply to the natural sciences. The characteristics of scientific enquiry can be summarized as follows.

Empiricism

For many scientists, a key feature of the scientific method is empiricism: a belief that scientific knowledge can only be derived from observable data. Such things as emotions, motives or inner meanings are thus not amenable to direct scientific examination. We can only research the empirical indicators of such phenomena (such as laughing, or particular actions).

Logical induction

Following on from the empirical approach is logical induction. This is the process by which theories, or laws, about the physical world are inferred from repeated empirical observations. An example of the inductive approach is research into the relationship between high blood pressure and stroke; repeated observation of a higher rate of stroke in people with high blood pressure leads to theories about the causes of stroke.

Realism

A key assumption for many scientists is that reality is stable, and exists outside our attempts to describe it. For example, a realist assumption is that there is a 'real' disease called malaria, caused by a plasmodium parasite, passed on by mosquitoes. It may be that in different historical times the causes of malaria have been differently understood (as the result of bad air, for instance) or that some sufferers may believe their malaria has been caused by evil spirits, or that the phenomenon is not a distinct disease at all and is simply an extreme version of other diseases such as 'flu. However, for the realist scientist, malaria is always a distinct disease with invariable causes, however we attempt to explain it.

Value-free nature of scientific enquiry

For many, science should exist outside the influences of society, such as religious, political or emotional views.

Together, the features characterize what is often called a *positivist* view of science. Positivism is a philosophy that holds that there are 'laws' governing the behaviour of the natural world and that the proper object of science is to discover them. To do this, scientists must study observable phenomena, which can be objectively measured. There have been many criticisms of the positivist view of science. We will come to them later in this chapter. However, positivism has had a significant influence on many social science methods, particularly the quantitative ones, so it is useful to start with an understanding of both positivism and the implications it has for scientific logic. Positivist social scientists attempt to study 'observable' facets or consequences of human behaviour, which can be measured, and attempt to derive general laws about behaviour from their observations.

Positivist social science – an example

In the social sciences, the work of the French sociologist Emile Durkheim (1858–1917) is often cited as an example of early positivist research. His study of records of suicide rates across Europe (Durkheim [1897] 1963) demonstrated that different societies had different 'propensities' to suicide: that individuals were more likely to kill themselves if, for instance, they lived in Protestant rather than Catholic societies, if economic conditions were poor, and if they were unmarried. From his analysis of suicide statistics, he developed a theory that linked the rate of suicide to a lack of social integration: when a community had close bonds, and individuals felt part of it, the suicide rate would be lower. Durkheim's findings are of less interest here than his approach, which illustrates the positivist tradition in social science.

✎ Activity 2.2

Why would you characterize Durkheim's approach to the study of suicide as a positivist one?

↻ Feedback

Durkheim used observable facts (recorded rates of suicide) rather than those that would have to be interpreted (such as motivations, or moral views) and he attempted to derive general laws from his data (that suicide rates vary with the level of social integration in a society).

Although few present-day researchers would describe themselves as 'positivist', positivism continues as an orientation of much social science, particularly quantitative social science, and it underpins the methodological approaches of many other health science disciplines.

However, there are a number of alternative approaches to scientific enquiry. These alternatives arise from two rather different kinds of criticisms of positivism:

- That the characteristics you read about do not really describe any kind of scientific research, even in the natural sciences. In this view, the characteristics are seen as either a simplistic, stereotypical description of how science works, or as a naïve view.
- That the characteristics you read about are *inappropriate* for researching questions to do with human behaviour, so positivism is an inadequate starting point for social scientific research.

A number of philosophers have taken the first of these positions: that it is naïve to assume that any kind of scientific research really progresses through the processes of empiricism and induction.

Is science really based on empiricism, induction, realism and value-free enquiry?

First, Karl Popper (1968), writing in the twentieth century, rejected the positivist view of scientific progress, suggesting that knowledge did not grow incrementally, by repeated observations to develop laws about the world, but by a more creative process that might include intuition, hunches, or inspiration. These creative processes generate *hypotheses* – provisional explanations for some aspect of the world. In a sense, it does not matter where initial hypotheses come from – what is important, is that they are tested. For Popper, a scientific law or theory can never be proved but it can be disproved. This model of scientific research is thus called the *hypothetico-deductive model*. The hypothesis is generated, and then tested through research, in order to try to falsify it. For Popper, it is the testability of hypotheses that characterizes scientific knowledge.

Alan Chalmers (1982) further argues that empiricism and naïve logical induction are not convincing as guarantors of the validity of scientific knowledge. Key to his critique is the logical impossibility of observing without presupposing a theory. However mundane our empirical observations, they require a set of expectations about the world and how it is for us to interpret them: we cannot 'see' (or use any other sense) without first having a theory (however low level) to frame what we are seeing. Thus, we can make repeated observations of the symptoms of malaria, but unless we have a pre-existing 'theory' of malaria, which distinguishes it from other causes of fever for instance, these observations will mean very little.

A third critique of the naïve positivist position comes from Thomas Kuhn (1962), whose ideas undermined a pure realist perspective. For Kuhn, scientific knowledge does not increase incrementally, but by radical changes in world views, which determine the kinds of questions scientists can ask and the theories they work with. He called these revolutionary changes *paradigm shifts*. The dominant paradigm of the day will shape what kinds of research can be carried out, in that anyone working outside the paradigm will find it very difficult to get their research funded or their results published. Paradigms shift as particular disciplines enter a 'crisis' mode, in which there are competing explanations, and existing theories cannot accommodate new knowledge that is generated. New paradigms emerge that can, for the moment, account for new knowledge. The implications of Kuhn's ideas are that science is a social process, in that research happens within a social world that is managed by elite scientists, and that explanations only make sense within a particular paradigm.

It is difficult when inside a paradigm to imagine science outside it: the dominant theories are so widely held that it would seem like nonsense to think outside them. However, it is perhaps a little easier to see the social influences on science. The kinds of research with which you feel driven to become involved, and that are funded and published, are inevitably shaped by influences outside those of science itself, particularly in areas like public health. Your own values, education, current national and local policies, the political needs of the communities you work with and the business activities of organizations such as drug companies will all shape the topics that it is possible to work on, and the kinds of questions you ask about those topics.

Relativist perspectives and the social sciences

There have, then, been a number of criticisms of positivism as a description of how scientific research happens. These have suggested that science is an activity rooted in society, and that social values will have an influence on what is researched and what kinds of answers we will find. More important, for a discussion of methodology, is that many social scientists believe that positivist approaches are inappropriate for research on human behaviour. Key for many of these criticisms is the rejection of realism. Instead of seeing reality as something that is unchanging and that pre-exists our attempts to research it, relativists believe that reality, and our knowledge of it, are 'socially constructed' in that they are a product of particular social, political and historical circumstances. Various kinds of relativist philosophy have had a major influence on social science methodology, particularly for the more qualitative traditions. When one adopts a particular relativist perspective on, for instance, illness, one accepts that other perspectives on it are equally legitimate. For instance, if we are studying the beliefs people with malaria have about how it is caused, we could treat beliefs such as 'it is a result of witchcraft' not as mistaken or ill educated, but as legitimate beliefs, if we understand the cultural perspective of those with this belief. This is not the same as 'agreeing' that malaria is caused by witchcraft but is a stance that says that this is a legitimate belief and that we can research it as such, rather than as a 'mistake'. This is a perspective known as cultural relativism, which is discussed further in Chapter 14.

A more extreme relativist position is that of *social constructivism*. For social constructivists, 'observable' facts (such as death rates, or symptoms of disease) are not objective facts, reflecting an underlying reality about the number of deaths from a disease, or the existence of disease in an individual. These labels merely reflect human attempts to categorize nature: there is nothing inevitable or natural about our definitions of such things as 'malaria' or 'a family' or 'virus'. Their meaning changes depending on how the reality is constructed. Symptoms of disease, for instance, are classified in different ways in different countries, and the category 'virus' only has a meaning within a particular biological theory.

Activity 2.3

How might a relativist criticize Durkheim's analysis of suicide rates?

Feedback

Relativist criticisms of Durkheim's analysis might include the following arguments. First, what we understand by 'suicide' is socially constructed and can change over time and from culture to culture. For example, the decision to not accept life-saving treatment for a fatal disease might be considered suicide by some people and not others. It is possible to imagine a future where death caused by tobacco smoking is considered 'suicide' (a deliberate action that leads to one's own death). Second, various social processes also 'construct' the recorded rate of suicide in a particular country. The actions of such officials as doctors, coroners and police officers are likely to be influenced by the very factors that Durkheim suggested influenced the rate of suicide. Thus, in a Catholic society, where the social stigma attached to suicide might be higher than in a Protestant country, there may be more incentive to record an accidental death in the same circumstances. Death rates reflect the ways in which deaths are recorded and classified, not any 'objective' reality about the number of deaths from different diseases.

You may also want to reflect at this point on your own assumptions about the world and your beliefs about how we can 'know' the world. Are you a 'positivist' who believes that there is a stable reality, which research should strive to represent, or are you a 'relativist' who believes that reality is constructed differently, depending on who is looking at it and from where? Many people have a shifting perspective, taking a more positivist position on some questions and a more relativist position on others. On suicide, for instance, they might accept that it is impossible to come up with an objective definition that would always represent the same 'reality' whereas they might feel more comfortable with the idea that there 'really is' a disease called malaria, which is always the same, irrespective of how it has been constructed in different times and places.

Interpretative approaches

Even if we accept a realist position, we may be more interested not in researching that reality but in researching people's *interpretations* of reality. For instance, if we are working in an area where people's understanding of malaria is very different to that of the dominant medical paradigm, the key research questions may be around *how* malaria is understood, rather than what malaria is. If we are interested, for instance, in changing people's health behaviour, what is important is an understanding of why they behave as they do and what their beliefs are. This is a principle of interpretative approaches to social research, where the aim is to understand the perspectives of those we are researching. Many qualitative researchers start from an interpretative approach, in that they are addressing questions about the *meaning* of reality (whether it is malaria symptoms, satisfaction with health services or the aims of a policy), rather than trying to determine what reality is. A key principle of this type of research is the acceptance that there is no one 'right' interpretation of meaning. For example, which definition of 'success' should we accept when judging the outcome of hip replacement: the patient's or the surgeon's? One might argues that patients have a more intimate understanding of their pain and quality of life or that surgeons are in a better position to compare a single patient with all the other patients that they have treated. However, we are no closer to proving that the one definition is more correct than another because we have no 'gold standard' of success to compare them with.

This chapter has provided an introduction to methodology, the general study of research methods and how they can produce valid knowledge about the world from different perspectives. In the next chapter we return to a practical issue concerning methods: how to frame a research question.

Summary

'Positivism' has been described as an approach to scientific research that assumes that reality is stable (is always the same, whoever is looking at it) and that research ought to measure observable features of that reality. In social sciences, there are alternative views. One is relativism, which in its extreme form assumes that reality changes and is constructed differently in different times and places. More common in health research are less strong versions of relativism, which assume that other perspectives on reality are worth studying to aid our understanding of people's health beliefs and behaviour.

References

Chalmers A (1982) *What Is This Thing Called Science?* (2nd edn). Milton Keynes: Open University Press.

Durkheim E [1897] (1963) *Suicide: A Study in Sociology*. London: Routledge & Kegan Paul.

Kuhn T (1962) *The Structure of Scientific Revolutions*. Chicago: University of Chicago Press.

Popper K (1968) *The Logic of Scientific Discovery*. London: Hutchinson.

Further reading

Chalmers A (1982) *What Is This Thing Called Science?* (2nd edn). Milton Keynes: Open University Press.

An accessible book for readers wanting to find out more about the philosophy of science. Chalmers looks at criticisms of science as observation and experiment, and at twentieth-century debates in the philosophy of science.

Smith MJ (1998) *Social Science in Question: Towards a Postdisciplinary Framework*. London: Sage.

This looks at how the social sciences have researched society, from the early influences of natural sciences models through to more contemporary perspectives.

3 | Framing a research question

Judith Green and John Browne

Overview

This chapter examines how broad topic areas of interest can generate more specific research questions. Good research questions are framed in appropriate terms so that it is clear how the research will answer them.

Learning objectives

After working through this chapter, you will be better able to:

- distinguish concepts, variables and indicators in research
- formulate research questions

Key terms

Concepts The phenomena that the researcher is interested in (such as 'inequalities in health' or 'social status'). These are not directly observable, but are assumed to exist because they give rise to measurable phenomena.

Indicators The empirical attributes of variables that can be observed and measured (such as 'blood pressure' or 'monthly wage').

Operationalizing The process of identifying the appropriate variables from concepts or constructs, and finding adequate and specific indicators of variables.

Variables Aspects of those phenomena that change (such as 'disease severity' or 'income').

From 'problems' to research questions

In Activity 1.3 you identified the kinds of problems that might be relevant to a health service manager and suggested that social science might have a role in providing research to inform solutions to those problems. But how do you turn the problems faced by the manager in that scenario into questions that can be researched rigorously?

One possibility: developing a hypothesis to test

One way of turning problems into research questions was suggested in the last chapter – think of provisional explanations for the observed phenomena and then develop 'falsifiable' hypotheses to test.

Activity 3.1

If you carried out a series of interviews with patients about their dissatisfaction with the service received from the department, one common answer might be 'I don't mind waiting, but I don't like not knowing how long I have to wait'. You want to carry out some research to find out whether telling people how long they will have to wait makes them less dissatisfied. What hypothesis would this study be testing?

Feedback

The hypothesis you suggested is likely to be along the following lines: 'patients who know how long the wait is will be less dissatisfied than those who do not know'.

We could then plan some research to test this hypothesis by, for instance, informing one group of patients of the likely wait and then distributing a questionnaire to compare their satisfaction with that of a control group, which was not informed.

Although it is sometimes possible in health research to frame a formal hypothesis of this sort, it is not always appropriate. It might not be appropriate because the question you need to answer is an *exploratory* one – the topic area could be one in which not enough is known to generate even a provisional explanation. One outcome of the research might then be to generate hypotheses as a result of the findings.

Activity 3.2

Think back to the accident and emergency department scenario in Activity 1.3 and specifically to the issue of junior doctors' treatment of the patients with minor problems.

1   Note down some of the reasons why junior doctors might investigate and treat these patients so intensively.
2   Why might we be interested in doctors' views?

↻ **Feedback**

> 1 Some reasons might include: need for practice in treating a range of health problems, uncertainty about how to treat minor illnesses, fear of missing a serious diagnosis, concern about litigation from dissatisfied patients.
>
> 2 Understanding why people behave as they do may suggest ways of changing that behaviour (for instance here it could be providing extra training, or support from senior staff) or may suggest that the behaviour cannot be altered in these circumstances and a new solution is needed. Here it might be providing other staff (perhaps nurses, or doctors with some experience of primary care) to treat patients with minor problems.

If we wanted to find out more about doctors' beliefs about their patients, and about their motivations to treat them intensively, we would not necessarily have a hypothesis to test. Rather, we would want to answer a more open question, such as 'Why do junior doctors intensively treat patients with minor illnesses?' Much qualitative research starts with these more open, exploratory questions, rather than formal hypotheses.

Concepts, variables and indicators

In social science research, then, not all questions can be framed as hypotheses. Sometimes research is focused more on understanding the nature of the concepts under study and how they relate to each other. In the social field this is often achieved by simply asking people questions or allowing them to tell their own stories, rather than attempting to control and intervene in the research context. Here, the question might be about understanding different perspectives, or exploring a topic to generate hypotheses. However, whatever the area of interest and the aim of the research, researchers must still frame their question in an appropriate way to answer it satisfactorily. In quantitative work, in particular, the process of developing a research question from a broad area of interest is sometimes called *operationalizing*. There are three stages that are typically involved:

Think about the concepts

First, think about the *concepts* you are interested in: the phenomena that are crucial to the problem. These are generally abstract constructs that have some theoretical meaning, but are hard to define exactly, such as equity, or social status, or occupational mobility, or health status. Concepts have many *dimensions*: health status, for instance, combines a number of factors, which might include life expectancy, presence or absence of symptoms, feelings of wellbeing, measures of physical strength or endurance, the intensity or severity of symptoms, and the relative importance of symptoms to the individual patient. Dimensions can be thought of as different aspects of the concept.

Identify the variables

The next stage is to separate out the different dimensions of the concept, and identify which of them are relevant to the research. These dimensions are the *variables* that will be used in the research: they should 'capture' something about the concept. A variable is a factor that changes (varies) in different circumstances, such as from individual to individual, or across time in the same individual. Thus, in Britain, 'social status' is a complex concept, often summed up by the term 'social class', which is hard to define precisely. For most it conjures up an interrelated set of factors, including people's income, their job, their educational level and aspects of their lifestyle. In other societies, the concept of social class may not be important at all, or may involve other dimensions such as religion, ethnicity, or caste. These dimensions of the concept are variables: they are not the same as the concept 'social class' but they do reflect one particular aspect of it. In Britain, the variables often used in research on social class and health are income levels and occupation. These are not identical to social class but they do reflect important aspects of it.

Decide on the indicators

Even though variables are more specific than concepts they are still not usually observable or 'measurable'. You cannot go out and 'measure' someone's occupation, or feelings of wellbeing. In quantitative research, variables themselves need operationalizing into empirical *indicators*, which can then be observed or 'measured' in the research. Indicators are operational level categories. For example:

- In a study of health status, the variable 'feelings of wellbeing' could be operationalized in terms of replies to questionnaire items such as 'How would you rate your own health for someone of your age group, on a scale of 1 to 5?'
- The variable 'occupation' could be operationalized as self-reports of primary occupation on a questionnaire.

Research questions in qualitative work

This process is perhaps easier to think about when the research question is framed as a hypothesis, or for quantitative research designs. However, even for exploratory questions, with the more 'open' research questions typical of qualitative work, it is still necessary to consider carefully how the question is framed. Thinking about the concepts involved is a useful exercise in ensuring that you have identified the most appropriate ones. Considering how you will gather empirical data to answer an exploratory question involves thinking carefully about what the evidence (the indicators) will be for those concepts. For instance, we suggested above the exploratory question: 'Why do junior doctors intensively treat patients with minor illnesses?' In thinking about how this will be answered, and perhaps reframed as a more specific research question, we need to consider the concepts of 'intensive treatment' and 'minor illness', as they may not mean the same things to the accident and emergency manager, the junior doctors and the researchers. We also need to consider how the 'why' question will be answered. Is this a question about doctors' motivations? In which case, what indicators will provide us with evidence about these 'motivations'? Or is it a question about how junior doctors make decisions about appropriate treatment? Thinking in detail about exactly what it is that the research will address will help refine the most feasible research question.

An example

Concepts, variables and indicators are not distinct: a particular category (such as health status) could be a concept in one context, but a variable in another. They can be thought of as being increasingly precise formulations. Formulating a research question involves specifying, as precisely as possible, the variables you are interested in and then identifying suitable indicators for them.

✎ Activity 3.3

Read the following extract, which summarizes the introduction to a 1994 paper by Henderson et al., on the utilization of health services in China. As you read, make notes identifying the concepts, variables and indicators mentioned. When you have finished, compare your notes with the feedback below.

Equity and the utilization of health services
This study investigated equity with respect to the provision and use of welfare services in eight Chinese provinces. In China, central government policies attempt to redistribute health resources to those in greatest need, but questions remain about whether services are available to those who need them. In an equitable system, individuals with similar health care problems will have equal access to health care, whatever their income level or other social attributes. In this study, a large sample of working-age adults who identified themselves as ill or injured in the four weeks prior to an interview was used to answer the question: 'What predicts use of health service for those sick or injured?' The researchers predicted first several predisposing factors (variables that influence the variable being studied) which would increase the use of health care services (including gender, occupation, educational level and age). Second was a range of enabling factors that were predicted to increase use. These included income, insurance levels and geographic location. Finally, they predicted that self-reported severity would be related to utilization.

In the survey, respondents were asked about the severity of their illness or injury; their experiences with the formal health care sector (although a large number also used folk healers); distance from the nearest health care facility, in terms of number of minutes taken by bike, and for a range of demographic information such as primary and secondary occupation, household income (including subsidies) and number of years in education.

↻ **Feedback**

The main concept used here is 'equity', which has been operationalized as 'equal access to health care for similar needs'. The variables the researchers are interested in include gender, occupation, educational level, age, income, insurance levels, geographic location, morbidity and severity, access to health care. Most variables have been operationalized as answers to a survey question, such as self-reports of use of formal health care; how many minutes it takes to cycle to the nearest health care facility and what the household income is.

This example shows that choice of indicator for a particular variable is a difficult task: no indicator is perfect. These researchers chose self-reports of illness or injury over the last four weeks and its severity as their indicator for 'need for health care'. These reports are relatively easy to collect compared with other indicators as respondents can be asked for the information, but other indicators could have logically (if not practically) been chosen.

✎ **Activity 3.4**

1 Can you think of any limitations of using self-reports of incidence and severity as an indicator for measuring 'need for health care'?
2 Which other indicators for 'need for health care' could you use in a population survey, if you wanted to study how equitable your health care system was?

↻ **Feedback**

1 Self-reports of severity are influenced by people's later health-seeking behaviour: if patients went to a secondary care facility rather than a primary health care clinic they may reconstruct the illness as more serious. Also, reporting behaviour is influenced by the very demographic variables that are being investigated, such as gender and educational level. Those people who are more likely to report the need for health care are not necessarily the same people who have more needs.

2 Other possible indicators include:

• mortality rates for different population groups
• time taken off work due to illness in a certain period
• self-reports of severe chronic illness
• measurements of markers for physical health, such as height, cholesterol levels, body mass index or low peak flow rates

Sometimes indicators are described as *proxy indicators* because they do not measure some aspect of the variable directly, but are known or assumed to be fair approximations for variables that cannot be measured directly. Thus self-reported weight can be used as a proxy indicator for clinician-measured weight, as there is a high correlation between the two measures. An example of a less exact proxy measure is postal district, which is often used as an indicator for the concept 'deprivation', even though it is obvious that there will be much variation in deprivation within the same postal area.

Whatever indicator is chosen, it will not be a perfect measure of the concept you want to research. Framing a research question involves some compromise, between what you would ideally like to know and what it is possible to measure. The possible indicators you may have thought of for 'need for health care' in Activity 3.4 may be more valid than those used by the researchers, but perhaps impossible to collect, or not feasible given the resource constraints of the project. The questions suggested in Activity 3.2 in Chapter 1, such as 'why do people attend the hospital with primary care problems?' are too vague to investigate as they are, but the process of turning them into researchable questions, with measurable indicators, compromises some of the meaning of the original concepts.

Activity 3.5

1 How would you frame 'Why do people attend the hospital for primary care problems?' as a researchable question?
2 Think about the main variables you would want to investigate, and list some possible indicators of them, which would be both appropriate and feasible to collect in a research study.

Feedback

1 First the different dimensions of the construct of 'primary care problems' need to be identified, in order to develop indicators that can be used in a research study. The other concept of interest is patient motivation: what factors influence patients' decisions to attend a hospital?

2 The table overleaf suggests one way of thinking about some possible variables for research; you may have developed others of relevance to the health care system you are familiar with, such as lack of health insurance or lack of appropriate primary care facilities.

Considering the concepts and possible indicators for them helps with the process of deciding exactly what to research, and what kind of data will be most appropriate to collect or generate. One outcome of the process suggested above for the research on those attending accident and emergency with minor problems might be deciding that a survey was needed to answer a research question about patients' motivations, such as: 'To what extent is lack of access to primary care a determinant of patients' decisions to attend the accident and emergency department with minor illness or injury?'

If enough is known already about some of the variables that are listed in the table it

Table 3.1 Why people attend hospital for primary care problems: refining concepts, variables and indicators

Concept	Possible variables	Possible indicators
Primary care problem	Minor illness or injury.	Patient left department without treatment Specific conditions identified in case notes.
	Problem treatable by primary care practitioner.	Triage nurse's assessment of problem. Doctor's assessment of problem.
	Duration of symptoms.	Onset of problem more than 48 hours ago.
Patient motivation to attend hospital	Dissatisfaction with local primary care facility.	Answer to questionnaire item on satisfaction with local primary care.
	Lack of access to primary care.	Answer to questionnaire item on availability of primary care. Availability of local primary care as recorded in official records.
	Inappropriate assessment of need for care.	Answers to case vignettes asking where you would go for treatment.

might be possible to move to a more formal hypothesis, such as: 'Patients attend accident and emergency departments with minor illnesses because they make inappropriate assessments of need for care'.

In Section 3 you will return to the design of quantitative research, including questionnaire surveys, which can address these sorts of questions. However, you may have noted that it is only possible to develop the kinds of variables in Table 3.1 if you already have some speculative theories about the problem. In the example discussed, such theories may, for instance, include the theory that lack of health insurance impacts on hospital use, or that patients and professionals have conflicting attitudes to the proper role of the accident and emergency department. These theories can come from professional experience, or from reviews of existing literature on the topic of interest. Often, though, these theories are at the level of untested 'common sense', or there may be conflicting accounts of possible explanations. When this is the case, a qualitative research study may be more appropriate. In the next section, you will examine the various kinds of qualitative methods that are used in health services research. First, though, there is a more general decision to take. Once we have refined a researchable question, and decided what *kind* of data might answer it (such as records from case notes, answers in interviews, blood pressure readings), we need to decide what kind of design is most appropriate for organizing these data. The next chapter introduces some common designs in social research.

Summary

Developing a good research question involves thinking about the concepts of interest, and which variables represent the important dimensions of that concept. A feasible quantitative research question must also define operational level indicators for those variables. For qualitative work, it is still helpful to think through what would provide evidence for the concepts you are interested in. In public health and health services research, choice of indicator is problematic and often involves a compromise between what is possible to collect and what adequately reflects the variables of interest.

References

Henderson G, Akin J, Zhiming L, Shuigao J, Haijiang M and Keyou G (1994) Equity and the utilisation of health services: report of an eight-province study of China. *Social Science and Medicine* 39: 687–700

Further reading

Mason J (1996) Planning and designing qualitative research, in Mason J (ed) *Qualitative Researching*. London: Sage

This chapter describes a very useful approach to developing and refining qualitative research questions, involving thinking through a series of questions about the research project and the nature of the phenomena to be investigated.

Miller DC and Salkind NJ (2002) *Handbook of Research Design and Social Measurement*. London: Sage.

4 Research design

Judith Green and John Browne

Overview

To answer a research question adequately we need to choose the most appropriate design: the best way to collect or generate the kind of data that are most likely to provide us with the answer to the question. A research design is more than just the data collection methods used (such as interviews or questionnaires) – it refers to the *logic* of how these data will be collected. There are a number of ways of thinking about the range of research designs used in the social sciences. Here we will introduce five common kinds of design used in qualitative and quantitative research: experiments, surveys, observational studies, documentary research and participatory research.

Learning objectives

When you have completed this chapter, you will be better able to:

- **identify the most appropriate research design for a particular research question**
- **identify the strengths and weaknesses of experiments, surveys and observational designs in the social sciences**

Key terms

Controlled experiment A research design in which outcomes in the experimental group are compared to those in a 'control' group.

Introduction

So far, you have seen that social research in health involves both qualitative and quantitative approaches, and a range of types of question, from formal hypotheses that can be tested to more exploratory questions. In thinking about appropriate indicators for the research you have to consider what kind of data will help you answer the research question. The next step is to think about the logic of the research: how the data are going to answer the question. Selecting an appropriate research design is essential for ensuring that your study is capable of answering your research question. Consider, for instance, the questions that might face a public health specialist who wanted to reduce smoking among the teenage population of a particular district. If planning a research programme to support this, they might want to know:

- How many teenagers smoke cigarettes regularly and are there particular sub-groups (such as girls, those in urban areas) who are more likely to smoke?
- Why do teenagers start smoking? Why do they stop?
- Would a health promotion campaign in schools be an effective way to stop teenagers taking up smoking?

The first is a *descriptive* question, which needs a design that can provide good data about the prevalence of smoking among particular groups. The second is a more *exploratory* question and would require a design that accessed the meanings smoking has for teenagers. The third is a question about *effectiveness*, and a design capable of addressing causal effects would be needed. Planning an appropriate research design involves thinking in detail about whether the kind of study you are proposing will generate the right kind of data to answer the research question you posed.

There are a number of ways of thinking about research designs and for considering the choices to be made between them. Here we introduce five common types of design (experiments, surveys, observational studies, documentary studies and participatory designs). This is certainly not an exhaustive list of study designs and (as we will see) it is not a perfect typology as many studies in practice will borrow elements of different designs and many will not fit neatly into any one of these formats. However, thinking about the particular strengths and weaknesses of these particular designs will suggest the issues that need to be considered in any project.

Experiments

In essence, an experiment is a study in which the aim is to compare phenomena before and after an intervention. In medical research, one commonly used experimental design is the *randomized controlled trial* (RCT). In an RCT, the key features are that those receiving the intervention (the 'experimental' group) are compared with those who do not (the 'control' group) and that participants are randomly allocated to either the control or experimental group. Experiments in general are strong designs for looking at research questions that are about cause and effect. Examples of such questions would be: 'Do bed nets sprayed with insecticide prevent more malaria infections than those without?' or 'Do exercise classes for elderly citizens reduce the incidence of falls for this age group?' These questions require a research design that enables us to see whether the intervention being tested (insecticide-treated bed nets, exercise classes) has a particular effect (reducing malaria or falls) in a particular population.

Activity 4.1

In a randomized controlled trial to investigate the effect of insecticide-treated bed nets, you randomly allocate 30 villages in your district to either the control group, which are given ordinary bed nets for each resident, or the experimental group, which are given treated bed nets. A nurse, who does not know which group the villages are in, visits each village each month to carry out household interviews to find out how many cases of malaria there have been. After a year, the incidence is much lower in the villages that have been given treated bed nets.

1   Why does this design enable us to be fairly confident that the intervention (treated
    bed nets) has caused the reduction in malaria, rather than other factors, such as
    higher use of prophylactics or a fall in the number of mosquitoes locally?
2   How do we know that the differences between the experimental and control vil-
    lages are not due to differences in the populations of those villages (such as numbers
    of children), rather than the interventions?
3   How do we know that the lower incidence in the experimental villages is not due to
    the nurse's bias (for instance, she is likely to expect fewer cases and thus be less
    likely to record them)?

↻ Feedback

1 Comparing the control and experimental group enables us to test the specific
contribution of the intervention, given that (in theory) the villagers should be subject to
the same other factors.

2 Randomly allocating villages to the two groups should, in principle, ensure that
differences are due to chance, and not any systematic differences that would influence
malaria incidence.

3 The nurse is 'blind' to whether the village has received the intervention or not.

Studies involving single interventions, such as new drugs, are relatively easy to
organize, at least in principle. In public health, however, we are usually interested
in more complex interventions such as health promotion campaigns or the introduction of new services. Even a relatively straightforward intervention, such as the
bed net in Activity 4.1, involves, in practice, a rather complex series of human
behaviours. Insecticide must be applied and paid for, the bed nets must be used
appropriately, villages may trade the bed nets between them, bed nets may be
taken out of the village by those who travel. In testing any complex intervention it
is much more difficult to answer a simple question about cause and effect because
we are often looking at complicated chains of causes, and at behaviour that is
embedded in everyday life rather than separated out in the laboratory. In health
services research, the term *pragmatic trial* is used to describe randomized controlled
trials in which the aim is to try to test these kinds of interventions in the 'real
world'. One example is an experiment that looked at whether additional social
support for pregnant women would improve outcomes for them and their babies.
The following is a summary of Ann Oakley's (1990) account of this trial.

A pragmatic trial of social support in pregnancy

There is a large research literature suggesting that social support is important for
women who are pregnant, and that those with little social support (from, for
instance, family and friends) experience poorer outcomes. The research team was
interested in whether a research intervention providing additional social support
could improve outcomes for women and their babies. An experimental design was

chosen to answer this question because previous research on this topic had been limited by potential confounding variables; it is impossible to say whether the better outcomes associated with better social support were really the result of social support, or just reflecting the fact that those with better social support are different in some way from those without. A randomized controlled trial (RCT) was planned that provided four midwives to visit women at home and offer emotional support. The population consisted of pregnant women who had previously given birth to a low birth-weight baby. Those consenting to being entered for the trial were randomly allocated to either receive this extra support or to be in the control group and receive normal maternity care only. Outcomes measured included women's satisfaction and birth weight.

Although an RCT is the strongest design for addressing the question about whether this kind of support does improve maternal and child outcomes, Oakley's account does illustrate the difficulties of organizing these kinds of pragmatic trials in real health service settings. Some of the problems she encountered were:

- Professionals are often uncomfortable about random allocation to services. If the midwives felt that women were in desperate need for social support, it was difficult for them knowing there was only a 50:50 chance of being allocated it. For professionals used to allocating services on the basis of perceived need, random allocation is difficult.
- Contamination. If participants are informed about a trial, many will want the potential benefits of the intervention. If they are not allocated to the experimental group they may try to get the same benefits in other ways, or may well talk to women they know in the other group.
- The conflicts between informed consent and rigourous testing. The research team were concerned to inform participants fully about the trial aims so they could make a decision about whether to take part. However, the more trial participants know about the study aims (for example that social support may improve satisfaction) the more likely it is that the outcomes will be biased.

A key issue for trials like this is *uncertainty*. It is only when we are genuinely uncertain of the benefits of an intervention that it is ethical to test it (otherwise, it would be unethical to withhold the intervention from the control group). However, 'uncertainty' may be difficult to agree on. Most medical interventions may never have been rigorously tested, yet it would not be ethical now to test them experimentally. In the case described here, many professionals believed that there was already enough evidence to suggest the benefits of social support and that an expensive RCT, which withheld the service for many in apparent need, was not needed. Oakley comments that genuine scepticism is very rare. However, experiments provide the only rigorous evidence we can have of whether something 'works' or not, and are likely to be much more convincing for policy makers.

Experiments are, then, a strong design for answering *causal questions*, when we need to be fairly confident that a particular intervention does have a particular effect in a given population. However, there are many reasons why this design may not be appropriate:

- First, not all questions are about causes. We may be more interested in describing some phenomenon, or exploring its meaning, than in determining what effects it has. A legitimate aim of much social science research is not predicting the effect of a variable or intervention (such as gender, or social support, or diagnosis) but understanding the meaning given to it by different participants. People, unlike the objects studied by natural scientists, reflect on their own behaviour (and on researchers' accounts of it) and change as a result. Research has to explore understanding as well as describing behaviour.

- A second limitation in much social research is that it may be impossible to separate out one particular intervention to study. In much health research you might be interested in examining the range of different factors that impact on behaviour, and how they interact, rather than just testing those that you predict will have an influence. Thus, if carrying out the study described in Activity 4.1, we might want to study such activities as bed-net trading, and how nets are used within households. Rather than being factors that 'interfere' with our research, these are the interesting aspects of behaviour that we need to understand in order to understand how bed nets are used in everyday life.
- Third, even if an experiment were the design of choice, it might not be possible for ethical or practical reasons. Imagine, for instance, that we were to hand out bed nets to only half of the villagers in a district. This might well cause resentment among the control villagers, and attempts to redistribute nets more fairly.

Activity 4.2

What other practical and ethical problems might be faced in carrying out the study described in Activity 4.1?

Feedback

A key ethical issue here is uncertainty. Given that there might already be good evidence that insecticide-treated bed nets are effective, some might consider it unnecessary to carry out a trial to test this. Gaining informed consent from all participants without jeopardizing the aims of the trial might also be difficult. If all villagers are informed of the aim (testing insecticide), they may ensure that all nets are treated, perhaps by buying insecticide to treat their nets from other outlets.

Surveys

A survey is a study design that collects the same data for each case in the sample. Examples include the censuses of the whole population, household surveys to collect data about family composition, or surveys of patients to evaluate their satisfaction with services. The issues to consider in designing and conducting a survey are discussed in Chapters 11 and 12, but these are some illustrations of the kinds of questions that surveys can address:

- Descriptive questions about population health and health behaviour. National surveys such as the General Household Survey in the UK collect data on health and health related issues (among other things) each year. These are invaluable data for such descriptive questions as: How many people smoke? How many men or women have limiting long-standing illnesses?

- Descriptive questions about public attitudes. Surveys are a useful way of taking a 'snapshot' of public attitudes or knowledge. One example is the European 'Eurobarometer', which, since 1974, has questioned people within each member state of the European Union to monitor social and political attitudes. This includes information useful for public health policy, such as public concerns about food safety, or trust in public information. Here we could use the data to answer comparative questions, such as where in Europe are consumers most concerned about the risks of food infection? However, comparing data across countries needs care and we need to be sure the instrument used has validity for the population. Surveys of attitudes are also used within health care organizations to look at users' perspectives.
- Studies of association. As well as descriptive analysis, we can use survey data to look at associations between different variables. Kaye Wellings *et al.* (1995), for instance, were interested in whether sex education in schools had an effect on the age at which young people first had sex. They used a national survey of sexual attitudes and lifestyles to look at associations between age at first intercourse and what kind of sex education they had received. They found men less likely to have had sexual intercourse before the age of 16 if they cited school as their main source of information about sexual matters.

The strengths of a survey design, if it is well planned and with a representative sample of the population of interest, is that they can generate good generalizable data. Well-designed surveys are in general good designs for descriptive research questions. If we can be sure that we have surveyed a representative sample of the population (see Chapter 12), with a reliable and valid instrument, we can be fairly confident that the results will be applicable to the whole population.

However, surveys cannot address questions about causation. To take the example above on the relationships between school-based sex education and age at first intercourse, we cannot conclude from the association that having school as the main source of education resulted in men delaying first intercourse, only that the two are related. It may be that men who had later first intercourse were just more likely to *report* school education as most important. If we need to look at causal relationships, ideally an experimental design is needed, if possible. In the case of sex education, this would be very difficult – we could not, for instance, deny sex education to a control group of young people and then compare their future sexual experiences. One alternative to experimental designs for addressing causal relationships is the *cohort study*, which repeats surveys of the same sample over time. Large cohort studies can look at how, for instance, health behaviour or social circumstances affect future health.

Observational designs

In the social sciences, an observational design is one that enables the researcher to observe behaviour in as 'natural' a setting as possible (note that it has a rather different meaning in epidemiology, where it would include cohort designs, which were mentioned above). In experiments, the researcher deliberately introduces an intervention. In surveys, the researcher asks for response to a predetermined set of questions. Observational designs are orientated towards describing and analysing everyday lives and behaviours. Traditional ethnographies in anthropology (see Chapter 14) are one example of observational studies, in which the researcher lives with those being studied for a long period of time in order to understand the world from their perspective. In more applied social research observational designs are often combined with other designs. For instance, we might use observational work at the beginning of a study to look at how a health care setting 'worked' before moving on to design an intervention study, or combine observations of meetings with interviews.

The key advantage of observational designs is that they allow researchers to answer questions about people's behaviour in everyday contexts: how people talk and act in their working and home lives. Ethnographic observational studies, if done well, can generate rich, deep information about one particular context. The disadvantage is that this is time consuming and we can usually only include one or a couple of sites within the study. They might then be limited in terms of generalizability.

Other kinds of observational design use 'naturally occurring' behaviour such as consultations in health care settings as the data. Here, audio or video recordings of consultations are transcribed in detail and analysed to answer questions about how health care providers and patients communicate. More quantitative approaches to observational data (such as counting the number of times nurses wash their hands on a hospital ward) resemble survey designs.

Documentary

The three designs discussed so far all involve collecting, or generating, new data. Documentary designs are those that use existing documentary resources as data. Modern organizations produce large numbers of documents: a hospital, for instance, produces medical and nursing notes on individual patients, summary reports of patient statistics such as numbers treated, management reports including statements of current strategies and annual reports, internal memoranda and emails between staff and possibly patient information leaflets or health promotion materials. Individuals also produce documents such as diaries and letters. Documents also include mass media such as newspapers, magazines and television programmes. There is, then, an enormous wealth of potential 'data' for health research that already exists. The following illustrates the way Henderson and colleagues (2000) used documentary sources.

The use of documentary sources: an example

Breast feeding rates in the UK are among the lowest in Europe. Lesley Henderson and colleagues were interested in how media images might create or reinforce ideas about breast and bottle feeding, and conducted a quantitative and qualitative analysis of how infant feeding was represented in the British media. They used two documentary sources of data: newspaper coverage in 13 national newspapers over one month, and television programmes including those directly relevant to health or infants, and a selection of news bulletins, soaps, medical dramas and advertisements over the same month. A quantitative content analysis of newspaper and television coverage identified how often references were made to breast and bottle feeding, in what context and whether any problems were associated with the method. The qualitative analysis was 'designed to explore the overall context and narrative in which the practice of infant feeding occurred'. This included analysing the language and imagery associated with breast or bottle feeding.

In the television coverage, they found that breast feeding was rarely shown. Most references to breast feeding were verbal, whereas references to bottle feeding were visual. When breast feeding was shown it was often associated with problems such as practical or emotional difficulties. No references were made to the health benefits of breast feeding. Again, newspaper coverage often commented on potential problems with breast feeding but rarely on its health benefits. This suggested that breast feeding was commonly associated with humorous story lines in fictional television programmes and with middle-class or celebrity women. In contrast, bottle feeding was presented as largely invisible and associated with 'normal' families. These documentary sources were, then, a source of information on how the media may play a role in perpetuating common ideas about breast feeding (that it is difficult and not something to do in public) and bottle feeding (that it is normal, and unproblematic).

Documentary designs have practical strengths. The use of existing documents can save time and money, if it is possible. Documents in the public domain, such as newspaper articles or reports of national statistics, are easily accessed. However, accessing documents such as medical records will require ethical approval and may be time consuming. Chapter 15, which introduces the discipline of history, looks in detail at some of the methodological issues raised by using documentary sources in historical studies. One key issue is that it is important to remember that documents cannot be used in any simplistic way as data about reality. In discussing how documents can be used in studies of organizations, Paul Atkinson and Amanda Coffey (1997) note that:

> . . . one must be quite clear what they can and cannot be used for. They are 'social facts', in that they are produced, shared and used in socially organized ways. They are not, however, transparent representations of organizational routines, decision-making process or medical diagnoses. They construct particular kinds of representations within their own conventions. We should not use documentary sources as surrogates for other kinds of data.

Participatory research designs

The final type of design to introduce is that of participatory research. For some researchers, the aim of research is not just to document or analyse the social world but to change it: this kind of research is often called *action research*. As Elizabeth Hart and Meg Bond (1995) note, action research 'may be particularly appropriate where problem-solving and improvement are on the agenda'. Participatory action research covers a number of perspectives, ranging from radical attempts at changing the social order through to more limited projects working on professional practice. Studies in these traditions include ambitious projects aiming at empowerment of rural villagers in developed country settings as well as smaller studies based on single hospital wards that are designed to improve nursing practice. What these perspectives share is a belief in research processes that include elements of working with (rather than researching on) participants in order for them to control the research agenda and outcomes and to identify desired changes. There is also usually an explicit commitment to viewing the knowledge of participants as essential to the process. Many studies in health include elements of participatory design. This can be at a minimal level of including representatives of user groups in steering committees (such as those from patients' associations) through to full participatory designs that attempt to redress radically the traditional power relationships within research. A short example of a participatory approach is described by Paine *et al.* (2002):

> The Stepping Stones project aims to empower communities to take control of their own sexual and emotional health. In evaluating the impact of Stepping Stones in the Gambia, the research team used a participatory approach that included the use of workshops with separate age and gender groups from the intervention villages. In these, villagers were invited to set priorities for action. Villagers changed the focus from 'family planning' to 'infertility prevention', in line with their own priorities about sexual health. Thus, rather than designing research using the agenda and priorities of the researchers, participatory approaches focus on changes identified by participants.

Other designs

The approaches we have suggested here are clearly not exhaustive, nor are they mutually exclusive. First, many projects include a number of designs used in sequence or in tandem (see Chapter 16). Also, individual studies may not 'fit' any of these designs. One example is that of the qualitative interview study, which is a little like a survey in that it collects data from a sample of individuals, but not the same data, and the data collected are not amenable to statistical analysis. Instead, the qualitative interview study utilizes some of the logic of naturalistic designs, in that the idea is to encourage respondents to talk 'as if' they were in naturalistic settings.

Research design and data collection methods

There is no inevitable relationship between the design of a study and the methods used to collect or generate data. Although experiments and surveys may be more associated with quantitative data collection methods, sometimes in-depth interviews or focus groups are used. In the trial of social support in pregnancy, the researchers used interviews to collect data post-intervention on women's views of the services they received. Similarly, an observational study could quantify observations. An example might be research on adverse events in a hospital ward. Although the design is observational, the researchers might want to classify particular events (drug errors, falls and so on) and count them. It is, then, important to *distinguish the design of the study and the data collection methods used.*

Summary

In this chapter, you have learnt about the importance of selecting an appropriate study design for the research question. Experiments are the strongest design for answering questions about causal relationships. However, they are not a common design in social research. First, there are often limitations on how far we can 'intervene' in human behaviour. Second, most of the research questions social researchers are interested in are not primarily about cause and effect but are about describing or understanding health and health-related behaviour. For these sorts of questions, surveys offer advantages for many descriptive questions, whereas observational designs may be strongest for questions reliant on in-depth understanding of human behaviour.

References

Atkinson P and Coffey A (1997) Analysing documentary realities, in Silverman D (ed) *Qualitative Research: Theory, Method and Practice*. London: Sage.

Hart E and Bond M (1995) *Action Research for Health and Social Care: A Guide to Practice*. Buckingham: Open University Press.

Henderson L, Kitzinger J and Green J (2000) Representing infant feeding: content analysis of British media portrayals of bottle feeding and breast feeding. *British Medical Journal* 321: 1196–8.

Oakley A (1990) Who's afraid of the randomized controlled trial?, in Roberts H (ed) *Women's Health Counts*. London: Routledge.

Paine K, Hart G, Jawo M, Ceesay S, Jallow M, Morison L, Walraven G, McAdam K and Shaw M (2002) 'Before we were sleeping, now we are awake': preliminary evaluation of the Stepping Stones sexual health programme in The Gambia. *African Journal of AIDS Research* 1. 41–52.

Wellings K, Wadsworth J, Johnson AM, Field J and Whitaker LB (1995) Provision of sex education and early sexual experience: the relation examined. *British Medical Journal* 311: 417–20.

Further reading

Cresswell JW (2002) *Research Design: Qualitative, Quantitative and Mixed Method Approaches* (2nd edn). London: Sage.

This is aimed mainly at postgraduate students planning a dissertation or thesis, but is a useful and readable guide to the steps in designing a proposal, from reviewing the literature through to writing it up in an appropriate way.

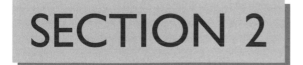

SECTION 2

Qualitative methods

5 | Introduction to qualitative methods

Judith Green

Overview

Traditionally, most of the research studies reported in academic journals in the area of public health are quantitative but there has been increasing interest in the contribution that qualitative studies can make. As well as adding to quantitative studies, qualitative ones can be used alone in research to address questions not amenable to experimental or survey research. Qualitative methods used in public health have their roots in the disciplines of sociology and anthropology. This section will introduce some of the methods used by sociologists and anthropologists and you will have an opportunity to explore how they can be used to address problems in health promotion, public health and health services management. Chapter 8 introduces some of the issues in analysing qualitative data, and Chapter 9 is a practical exercise designed to give you some experience in using qualitative methods.

Studying Chapters 5 to 9 will enable you to identify some of the different perspectives in qualitative health research and to identify the advantages and disadvantages of qualitative interviews and focus groups as qualitative data-collection methods, and will help you to understand the range of methods used to analyse qualitative data.

Learning objectives

After working through this chapter, you will be better able to:

- identify the main aims of qualitative research designs
- identify appropriate research questions for qualitative designs

Key terms

Interpretative approaches Those that focus on understanding human behaviour from the perspective of those being studied.

Naturalism Studying social behaviour in the context in which it 'naturally' occurs.

What are qualitative methods?

Qualitative methods are characterized as those that aim to explore meaning and that produce non-numerical data. Qualitative data can be produced by a range of data-collection techniques. These include:

- *participant observation* in which the researcher participates, to some extent, with the group he or she is studying
- *in-depth interviewing* to explore the attitudes and experiences of individuals
- *focus groups* or group interviews
- *audio-taping naturally occurring talk*, such as consultations between health professionals and patients
- *analysing textual or pictorial data*, such as diaries or photographs, to explore what they can tell us about the individuals or societies that produced them.

However, these data-collection techniques can also produce quantitative data. Participant observation could, for instance, be designed to quantify aspects of human behaviour, such as counting the number of times nurses speak to patients, or the number of questions patients ask in a consultation. Similarly, textual data (diaries, magazine articles, newspaper reports) could be quantitatively analysed by counting the number of times a concept is mentioned, or the number of column inches devoted to a topic.

What makes a research design qualitative is not the data-collection strategy used, but the aim of the study and how the data produced are analysed. Health care research using qualitative techniques has a range of different aims, but common ones include those of *understanding* the experiences and attitudes of patients, the community or health care workers. In public health research, this is often done with the goal of informing policy makers or practitioners. In an article arguing for the greater use of qualitative methods for assessing health care, for instance, Ray Fitzpatrick and Mary Boulton (1994) summarize their view of the aims of qualitative research:

> Qualitative research depends upon not numerical but conceptual analysis and presentation. It is used where it is important to understand the meaning and interpretation of human social arrangements such as hospitals, clinics, forms of management, or decision making. Qualitative methods are intended to convey to policy makers the experiences of individuals, groups, and organisations who may be affected by policies.

In this chapter, you will examine the aims and potential uses of qualitative methods in more detail before going on to look at the discipline of medical anthropology and at two specific qualitative research techniques: qualitative interviewing and focus groups in subsequent chapters. These data-collection techniques may seem diverse but they do have some basic orientations towards research in common, apart from their tendency to produce language, rather than numerical data.

Orientations of qualitative research

Many qualitative researchers share a set of assumptions about the research process, including the aims of research and how research ought to proceed. Three of these orientations are outlined here. They are an interpretative approach, a commitment to naturalism and the adoption of flexible research strategies. Of course, not all qualitative studies or researchers will feature these orientations at all times.

Interpretation

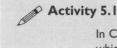

Activity 5.1

In Chapter 2, two alternative views of research were outlined: the positivist position, which assumes that there is one stable reality to be uncovered in research, and the relativist position, which assumes that there are many possible realities, which are constructed (in part at least) through social action. Which of these two positions do you think best characterizes qualitative research?

Feedback

Much qualitative research has a relativist starting point. As the aim is to explore how people understand events and phenomena, researchers start by assuming that there are different possible and legitimate understandings.

Qualitative social researchers are interested in multiple social realities and they try to avoid assuming that their view of the world is the only valid and rational one. Thus what appears common sense to one social actor may not be to another. A good example of this is research on lay health beliefs – which to the professional may appear irrational and unscientific but which have a consistency and rationality for the patient and may lead to very different ways of conceptual-izing health and disease from those of health professionals. Interpretative approaches start from the assumption that if you come to understand how respondents see the world then you will understand the logic and rationale behind what might at first seem bizarre beliefs or behaviours. This is sometimes called an *interpretative approach* in that it aims to interpret how people conceptualize the world. The orientation towards interpretation and understanding is illustrated by the work of the American sociologist Erving Goffman. In a study of large psychiatric institutions, he used participant observation to understand the lives of patients who lived in them and staff who worked there (Goffman 1961). He wrote of the importance of seeing the world through the eyes of those being studied:

> any group of persons develop a life of their own that becomes meaningful, reasonable and normal once you get close to it and a good way to learn about any of these worlds is to submit oneself in the company of the members to the daily round of petty contingencies to which they are subject.

In contrast to positivist social science, where only 'observable' phenomena are of interest, interpretative social science also studies non-observable phenomena, such as the meaning people attribute to their behaviour.

Naturalism

A second orientation of many qualitative studies is a commitment to *naturalism* – the importance of trying to study action in its natural context rather than, for instance, in the laboratory or in terms of answers to questionnaires. What people say and do is related to where they are – action is contextual. People take medications in their home, when out, to fit in with the rest of their lives, not in the controlled conditions of the drug trial. Health workers relate to their clients in hospitals, clinics and in clients' homes, not in their offices where they fill in your survey questionnaires. One of the advantages of qualitative research is that it can inform practitioners and policy makers about how policies are put into practice (or not) in 'real life'. A summary of a study of asthma patients in the UK by Adams and colleagues (1997), illustrates this.

Using qualitative research: an example

Stephanie Adams, Roisin Pill and Alan Jones were interested in the general problem of 'why patients do or do not take their medication as prescribed' (1997: 1) and how qualitative research can contribute to our understanding of how decisions that might seem irrational (such as not taking prescribed medication) can be understood better by taking a patient-centred perspective. Asthma is a common condition, and from the perspective of health professionals, poor compliance with prophylactic medication (the 'preventer' inhaler) and over-use of the 'reliever' inhaler (intended only for relieving symptoms) contributes to high rates of morbidity and mortality. Adams and colleagues used in-depth interviews with 30 patients to understand behaviour from the patients' perspective.

When they analysed the interviews, the researchers identified three broad patterns of response to asthma diagnosis and symptoms. For about half the sample, 'denial' or 'distancing' characterized their accounts. Most denied that they had asthma, preferring to describe themselves as having chest trouble or short-term conditions. Although denying they had asthma, detailed stories from their interviews suggested that their symptoms did interfere with everyday life, entailing avoidance of exercise or of going outdoors on occasion. This group also hid their medication use to a large extent, reporting using inhalers only out of sight of others, and had negative views of asthmatics – an identity they did not accept for themselves. Most did not use preventative medications at all – partly because of worry that they would become dependant on drugs that have to be taken daily, but also because taking medication regularly, whether there are symptoms or not, relies on accepting an asthmatic identity, which these 'deniers' did not. Given that they didn't see themselves as having asthma, they did not attend special clinics for asthma.

A smaller group within the sample accepted both the diagnosis and their doctors' advice completely, using medications as prescribed and taking pride in doing so. For this group, the route to 'normal life' was gaining adequate control over symptoms through medication. Their definitions of asthma coincided with those of medical professionals. For them, 'asthmatic' was not a stigmatized identity, and they used inhalers in public.

The final response was identified among a few respondents, described as 'pragmatists'. This group did use preventative medication, usually not as pre-scribed, however, but only when their asthma was particularly bad. They also had a pragmatic approach to disclosing asthma diagnosis, for instance, in telling family, but not employers in case it prejudiced their employment prospects. This group accepted they had asthma, but usually perceived it as mild, or as an acute rather than chronic illness.

Looking at medication use from the point of view of patients enabled the researchers to see how health behaviour was tied tightly to people's beliefs about asthma and what kind of chest problems they had, as well as social circumstances and the threat of an asthmatic identity to other social identities. For patients, health, defined in medical terms, may not be the top priority all the time, and the meaning of symptoms for professionals may be rather different from the meaning of symptoms for patients.

Activity 5.2

How might these findings be useful to primary care practitioners who are planning a special asthma clinic in their practice?

Feedback

For service providers and health promoters this kind of information is very useful. First it suggests that providing designated asthma clinics may not appeal to the majority of sufferers, either because they do not identify themselves as having asthma or because they see themselves as in control of their condition. Second, professionals can see that what appears to be irrational use of medication and the result of ignorance is actually deeply embedded in complex social identities that have to be managed.

Flexible research strategy

A third orientation of qualitative research is the adoption of a flexible or 'open' research strategy. Quantitative studies tend to follow standardized research stages, which are reproduced when writing up for publication. Studies start per-haps with the definition of a hypothesis to test, then proceed to designing a data-collection instrument, collecting the data, and then analysing data to produce results. This is, of course, a proper way to proceed if there is a firm hypothesis to test. However, in qualitative studies the research question may be informed by the priorities and experiences of participants such as interviewees, and become refined as a result of early data collection and analysis. Analysis starts as soon as data are collected, rather than at the end of the study. This initial analysis can also inform later sampling. This is known as *theoretical sampling*, when cases or sites are included in the study on the basis of an emerging theory about relationships between variables rather than as a result of an initial, one-off sampling decision.

When is it appropriate to use qualitative methods?

Before we can count events or phenomena in a quantitative study, we have to know what *should* be counted: what the relevant variables are and how they should be defined to inform the researchers about the concepts they are interested in. Qualitative work is an important part of this, especially if the research topic is a relatively new one. In this situation, qualitative research can help generate hypotheses, which can later be tested using more quantitative designs. Qualitative designs are useful for generating theory, and developing new concepts. At a more practical level, qualitative work is essential in questionnaire design to ensure that the phrases and language used are meaningful ones for those who will be completing the questionnaire.

However, qualitative methods are not just a precursor of quantitative designs. They can also answer questions not amenable to experimental or other methods. The following is a summary of a research study by Marion Gantley and colleagues (1999), which shows how qualitative research can illuminate quantitative findings: in this case the finding that ethnicity is related to rates of sudden infant death syndrome.

Using ethnographic methods: an example

Sudden infant death syndrome is the most important cause of death for infants aged between 1 and 12 months in the UK. The rate varies across the different ethnic groups that make up the UK population, with babies born to mothers from Bangladesh having significantly lower rates that those born to mothers born in the UK, Northern Ireland or the Caribbean. Epidemiological evidence and current knowledge about risk factors does not help explain this difference, and the researchers were interested in whether infant care practices might contribute to this low rate. To investigate infant care practices, they undertook a qualitative study in which they asked parents to describe a day in the life of their infant. They interviewed mothers who were born either in south Wales or Bangladesh who had children under 1 year old.

From these interviews, they identified some themes that suggested some differences in the ways in which infant care happened in Bangladeshi or Welsh households. First, in the Bangladeshi households, infants were more likely to be in households where childcare was shared between a number of adults, such as brothers and their wives living together in extended families, whereas the mothers born in Wales were more likely to be in nuclear households with just parents and their children. Second, extended families of cousins and grandparents meant that people other than parents were more likely to be involved with childcare than in the Welsh households. Bangladeshi families were more likely to have larger numbers of children, meaning there was more general familiarity with infant care. For the Welsh mothers, the arrival of a child was more likely to lead to dramatic changes in lifestyle. Welsh mothers were more likely to focus on regularity and routine in household management and infant care, in contrast to Bangaldeshi mothers who stressed fluidity and flexibility. Bangladeshi infants sleep close to other people, but Welsh mothers felt it important to get babies used to sleeping alone, in their own cots at first, and in their own rooms where this was possible.

It is not possible from this kind of study to identify which practices might protect against sudden infant death, but the findings do suggest some useful pointers to explore potential physiological mechanisms, such as the sensory stimulation from others that might help regulate breathing for human infants.

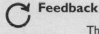 **Activity 5.3**

Why do you think the researchers used a qualitative design for this study?

Feedback

They were interested in the broad area of 'infant care practices', and wanted to explore differences between two ethnic groups in the UK. Not enough was known about how these might affect child health to develop either a structured survey, or to start testing cause and effect. Qualitative designs are particularly useful for these kinds of exploratory questions.

Summary

Qualitative methods aim to focus on how people interpret their social worlds and to explore the meaning of phenomena and events for participants. They contribute to health and health services research by investigating issues not amenable to quantitative analysis, by informing the development of quantitative tools and by exploring the processes described by statistical research.

References

Adams S, Pill R and Jones A (1997) Medication, chronic illness and identity: the perspectives of people with asthma. *Social Science and Medicine* 45: 189–201.

Fitzpatrick R and Boulton M (1994) Qualitative methods for assessing health care. *Quality in Health* 3: 107–13.

Gantley M, Davies DP, Murcott A (1999) Sudden infant death syndrome: links with infant care practices. *British Medical Journal* 306: 16–20.

Goffman E (1961) *Asylums*. Harmondsworth: Penguin.

Further reading

Green J and Thorogood N (2004) *Qualitative Methods for Health Research*. London: Sage.

This introduction to qualitative methods is aimed at health professionals who need to use qualitative findings or conduct their own studies, and introduces key issues in research design, data collection and analysis. It uses examples from a range of health care systems.

Qualitative interviewing

Judith Green

Overview

Qualitative interviewing involves using a semi- or unstructured topic guide to explore how respondents experience, conceptualize or construct their social worlds. This method has been widely used in health research to explore the beliefs and views of users and providers of health care.

Learning objectives

After studying this chapter, you will be able to:

- identify the uses of qualitative interviewing
- develop your skills in designing topic guides
- develop your skills in asking questions and listening to answers

Key terms

In-depth interviews The interviewer uses a topic list but respondents' priorities influence the final range of questions covered.

Rapport Relaxed, natural communication between interviewer and respondent.

Semi-structured interviews The interviewer uses a guide in which set questions are covered, but can prompt for more information.

Structured interviews The interviewer uses a schedule in which questions are read out in a predetermined order.

Research interview methods

Interviewing is one of the most commonly used methods in social research in health, and qualitative (or in-depth) interviews are only one type of research interview. Table 6.1 illustrates one typology of interviews, where they are classified by how *structured* they are, or the extent to which the questions asked by the researcher are predetermined.

Many surveys, especially those aiming to generate data that are generalizable to the whole population, favour the use of standardized interview formats, where the same questions are asked in the same order of each respondent, and the interviewers' job is to be as neutral as possible, so they do not influence, or bias, the

Table 6.1 Types of interview

	Format of questions	Example of uses
Structured	Standardized, predetermined, asked in the same order	Survey research
Semi-structured	List of questions or interviewer prompts	Surveys or qualitative studies
In-depth (sometimes called *narrative* or *qualitative*)	Broad topic guide	Qualitative study

respondents' answers. This is more likely to produce standardized data amenable to statistical analysis. In these kinds of surveys, if interviewers are used, they are, in effect, a tool for collecting responses, and interaction between interviewer and respondent is seen as a problem to be managed – it potentially interferes with reliability. From the more positivist perspective, the aim is to minimize the influence that interviewers have on the data they collect – to remove, as far as possible, interviewer bias. We will return to standardized, or structured, interviews in Chapters 10 to 13, when survey research is introduced.

In qualitative approaches, researchers are more likely to start with other assumptions about the nature of an interview, the status of data collected and the role of the interviewer. The role of the interviewer shifts depending on the perspective employed in the research. The qualitative interview provides a method of gaining in-depth information about people's beliefs and interpretations of the world.

In qualitative work, interviews are therefore more commonly *semi-structured* (with a set of questions to cover, but which can be rephrased to suit the understanding and vocabulary of the respondent, and which can be probed for more information), or *unstructured*. You will see a number of different terms to describe unstructured interviews, such as qualitative interviews and narrative interviews. These terms generally refer to interviews in which the interviewer has a list of prompts or topics to focus the interview but the conversation is guided by the priorities of the respondent. The advantage of using semi-structured approaches is that similar data can be gathered from all respondents; the advantage of using unstructured interviews is that they are more likely to elicit the views and priorities of the respondents rather than merely gathering their responses to the researcher's concerns. The best approach to use depends on the aims of the research. When it is important to explore in detail the respondents' own perceptions and accounts, a less structured approach will be most useful. This might be the case if researching a topic on which little is known, or when it is important to gain an in-depth understanding of a topic.

What makes a good qualitative interview?

Qualitative interviewing requires perhaps rather different skills on the part of interviewer from those required for more structured interviewing. Both kinds of interviewer need social skills in putting the respondent at ease, so that trust is established, and they feel comfortable in talking about experiences and attitudes.

This is known as good rapport. In qualitative interviews, often the aim is to recreate the flow of a 'natural' conversation, which requires additional skills in listening and asking appropriate questions. The interviewer must be able to listen attentively without appearing judgemental, and use prompts and probes appropriately and sensitively to lead respondents to expand on their ideas. Interviews in qualitative research are usually tape-recorded and then fully transcribed, both to allow a good rapport to develop between interviewer and respondent, and to allow full analysis of the interview based on the respondent's real words. This can be time consuming: one hour of taped conversation can take five hours to transcribe fully.

Qualitative interview topic guides

A key element of a good interview is developing the right questions to ask. Even if using less structured approaches, it is worth spending some time on thinking about the best ways to elicit the most useful data for your research question. Your respondents (whether they are patients or professionals) are unlikely to share your perspectives on the world, your classifications, or your vocabulary, so you need to develop questions that allow them to frame appropriate answers.

Activity 6.1

A hospital psychiatric department is concerned at the high drop-out rate from its treatment programmes. You want to interview people who have been diagnosed with schizophrenia, but who have not returned to the clinic, to see what their perceptions are of their disease and what kind of help they think the hospital can provide for them. The first two questions on your proposed topic guide are:

'How has schizophrenia affected your life?'
'Why have you dropped out of the hospital treatment programme?'

Why might these not work very well at establishing rapport or eliciting useful information?

Feedback

First, patients may not share the interviewer's classification of their diagnosis. It might be better to elicit first how patients think about their (mental) health problems, rather than using a medical diagnosis. Look back at the example in Chapter 5 on exploring patients' understanding of asthma if this is not clear: the researchers in this example found that many people who had been diagnosed with asthma did not share this view of their 'chest troubles'. The second question again uses the researcher's frame of reference: that 'dropping out' is a problem and that the interviewee can account for it as a 'problem'. It would be more useful to ask about views of hospital treatment in a more neutral way by, for instance, asking about what interviewees' expectations were of treatment, and whether they had been met.

One temptation is always to simply ask interviewees our research question, but this is rarely a useful question to ask directly in an interview. For instance, the following are reasonable questions for researchers to consider, but neither would generate useful information if asked directly of an interviewee:

'Is poor knowledge about malaria transmission a barrier to using bed nets in this village?'
'Is inappropriate antibiotic prescribing the result of doctors being unaware of current guidelines?'

It is not just that these questions use vocabulary that might be unfamiliar. More importantly, they would merely generate respondents' views about your research question, which is not the intention. In an interview you want to generate data that, when analysed, will answer your research question – not generate a list of rather superficial thoughts on the answer to that question. So, how can we ask questions that are likely to generate useful data? There are no hard-and-fast rules on how to do this. You need to think first very carefully about what kind of data will be useful. If we are interested in why villagers do not use bed nets, we might want to start by generating lists of all the possible causes of malaria, from their perspectives, or talk more generally about what they think about bed nets and how they are used. If we want to understand why doctors prescribe antibiotics 'inappropriately' it may be more useful to ask questions that generate data on why and in what circumstances they prescribe. You need then to think about what kinds of questions generally elicit these kinds of data from the people who want to interview. Direct simple questions sometimes work, but often we need to think more imaginatively.

Rules of thumb for asking interview questions

- Start with *general* questions. To begin, use a general question both to orientate your interviewees to the topic, and to elicit the kind of language they prefer to use. For instance, 'Tell me about how you came to be a patient in this hospital' or 'Can you start by telling me a bit about your working day here as a nurse?'
- Ask *open* questions. These are questions that require more than a 'yes' or 'no' in answer.
- Ask *neutral* questions. Instead of 'Why haven't you had your children immunized?' ask 'How did you make the decision about whether to immunize your children or not?'
- Use *appropriate everyday vocabulary* not medical terminology. Ask about 'your heart trouble' not 'your ischeamic heart disease', for instance.
- Use *concrete* rather than *abstract* questions. Talking about specific incidents rather than abstract ones is often easier. So instead of asking 'What do you like and dislike about maternity services?' ask 'Think about last time you were pregnant. What did you like about the services you received then?'

Sometimes we need to think more imaginatively about how to elicit particular kinds of information. Knowledge is sometimes difficult to access and tied to particular contexts. Here are some suggestions of types of question that can be used as alternatives to simple questions:

- *Diary questions*. Asking people to describe 'a day in their life' or 'a typical shift at work' can be a useful way to both introduce a topic, and to elicit what is important to them to talk about.

- *Critical incidents*. Asking about the best or worst experience they have had may be a useful way to elicit what is important to them about a topic. For instance, asking about 'the best dentist you ever had' and asking why might be more productive in generating data about what people think are important criteria for 'good dentists' than asking directly 'What do you think makes a good dentist?'
- *Free listing*. This can be useful in more structured interviews, and involves asking people to list all the examples they can think of in a certain category, such as all the possible causes of malaria, or all the possible treatments they use for fever in children.
- *Ranking*. Interviewees can be asked to rank items generated by free listing in order of importance, or efficacy.

Developing rapport

The sociologist Richard Sennett (2003), in reflecting on his early experiences as a field researcher, describes how he came to develop interview skills:

> In-depth interviewing is a distinctive, often frustrating craft. Unlike a pollster asking questions, the in-depth interviewer wants to probe the responses people give. To probe, the interviewer cannot be stonily impersonal: he or she has to give something of himself or herself in order to merit an open response. Yet the conversation lists in one direction; the point is not to talk the way friends do . . . The craft consists in calibrating social distances without making the subject feel like an insect under the microscope.

This reflection suggests both that interviewing is a craft – the skills needed can be developed through practice – and that it requires some insight into the appropriate relationship with the interviewee. The development of a good relationship is referred to as 'rapport': the establishment of a relaxed interchange in which inter-viewees feel able to talk without feeling judged and have the space to tell their story. This is a skill that builds on the techniques we use in everyday life to listen to the stories and opinions of others, although, as Sennett notes, it is not quite like the kind of interchange you might have with your friends. First, the conversation is more directed in that you are trying to elicit talk on a more-or-less defined topic. Second, the aim is usually not for you to expound your opinions and beliefs as well, but solely to elicit those of your interviewee.

The interviewer must be aware of cultural and social differences, not because these should be eliminated but because they need to be taken into account in qualitative work. Often we are interviewing people from very different backgrounds: from different professions, genders, ethnicities, ages or social status. These differences have an effect on all aspects of the interview: how likely it is that someone will agree to be interviewed, how much they feel they can disclose, how they frame their answers to your questions. On some very sensitive topics it might be sensible to 'match' interviewers with interviewees in terms of characteristics such as ethnicity or gender.

Although we cannot change our social characteristics, we can adopt the kinds of behaviour that are more likely to engender rapport. The specific behaviours will differ from setting to setting, and on what the normal 'rules' for interaction are in the setting in which you are working. In general, though, the key is to appear interested, non-judgemental and encouraging. So if you want, for instance, to probe your respondent on an unusual opinion, or extreme view, don't look surprised or disapproving, but perhaps probe with some more neutral questions:

'Do you think that is a view shared by most people?'
'Other people might think X: what would you say to them?'

To maintain rapport in an interview, the interviewer needs to listen carefully to answers so that the next question follows on and so that respondents don't have to repeat themselves. Some of the ways in which this is achieved will include:

- Eye contact. In many cultures, it is important to maintain eye contact, but without staring at the interviewee.
- Making the appropriate non-verbal noises or prompts (such as 'um-hm', 'yes', 'um' in English) and nods of encouragement that make people feel they are being listened to and can carry on speaking.
- Following up points where appropriate, or making appropriate comments in response ('that sounds difficult', 'was anything else important?').
- Not interrupting. This is often difficult to start with, as interviewers can be anxious not to leave a long space in the conversation, or to continue through the topic guide.
- Not giving our own opinions or disagreeing.

Nicky Britten (1995) notes that those experienced in clinical interviewing already have some of the skills needed to be a good qualitative interview but these skills do need adapting to generate good data from in-depth interviews, rather than clinical history-taking interviews:

> To achieve the transition from consultation to research interview, clinical researchers need to monitor their own interviewing technique, critically appraising tape recordings of their interviews and asking others for their comments. The novice interviewer needs to notice how directive he or she is being, whether leading questions are being asked, whether cues are picked up or ignored, and whether interviewees are being given enough time to explain what they mean. (1995: 252)

The general context of the interview will also have an effect on the kind of data you obtain. People talk differently in 'private' space (such as their home) than they do in public spaces (such as their workplace) and as you get to know people they are more likely to disclose less socially acceptable views and experiences. Jocelyn Cornwell (1984), in her study of people's accounts of health and illness in east London, interviewed her participants at different points, and she noted that in early interviews they gave different explanations and stories than in later ones, when they trusted her more as a friend rather than an 'outsider'. She called these accounts 'public' and 'private' accounts. It is not that the 'private' accounts are more accurate, or that her interviewees were lying in the more public, earlier ones, but just that people frame their responses differently in different contexts.

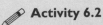

Activity 6.2

A team of primary care physicians want to find out what their patients think of the family planning services they offer from their practice, and what their understanding is of various contraceptives available. They plan to interview patients in the waiting room as they are waiting to see the clinic nurse. What comments would you have on the kind of data they are likely to generate?

Feedback

Patients may be very reluctant to disclose their negative views of services to those who are clearly clinic staff. They also may be inhibited by talking in a medical setting, particularly if there is no private space. If the interviewers are hoping to access more 'personal' accounts of understanding, they may need to interview patients in their homes, and perhaps match by gender. If more private accounts are needed, which might be a better guide to patients' behaviour, they may need to do repeat interviews.

How can qualitative interviews contribute to understanding health care?

Chapter 14 introduces the discipline of medical anthropology as one of the social science disciplines that explore health and health-seeking behaviour. Anthropology uses a number of methods of data collection, including observational methods and interview methods. Traditional anthropological studies used long-term participant observation to produce in-depth ethnographies of particular settings – although applied medical anthropology often uses more focused and less time-consuming approaches. In sociological studies it is more common to rely on interviews as the primary method of collecting data. While this has the potential to produce useful and rich data on perceptions and world views, there are limits to how far we can use interview data as a good guide to behaviour. This section considers interviews as a method for providing insight into how organizations are perceived by those who work within them, and how their 'talk' helps to construct organization. The structures that deliver health care – hospitals, the division of health care labour, the family (within which decisions about seeking health care are made, for instance) – are in part made real by the ways in which they are talked about: what it is possible to say, and in what contexts it is said. The following is an example of one research study that took this approach, in looking at how managers' talk contributed to the effectiveness of hospital organization (Green and Armstrong 1993, 1995).

Bed management: a qualitative study

Many London hospitals experience problems in finding enough in-patient beds for admitting emergency patients. One solution examined in this study was the introduction of 'bed managers' in nine London hospitals. These were designated managers who monitored and controlled access to beds across the hospital, in all specialties and wards, in order to make maximum use of the resources available and to balance the needs of emergency patients and those booked for elective surgery. In some hospitals these managers appeared to have successfully achieved authority over areas that were traditionally seen as areas of clinical decision making, such as the decision to admit or discharge a patient, or to place a patient on a particular ward. The researchers used semi-structured interviews with senior nurses, clinicians and managers, in which a topic list included questions on respondents' perceptions of the problem of emergency admissions and their experience of responses to it. They also used observation of the work of the bed managers. The researchers found a high level of consensus about the success of bed management. How had these managers achieved this, given the traditional conflict between clinical and managerial authority within hospital organization? Analysis of the interview data suggested that there were three 'rhetorics' used by bed managers, which contributed to their successful presentation of management as the solution to the problem (rather than more resources, for instance). The first of these rhetorics was that of a 'constant crisis', as illustrated by this comment from an interview with a bed manager: 'I mean, it's crisis management all the time and bed management won't be anything else unless there is no casualty, no emergency services, no referrals from GPs – it's always going to be crisis management'.

Staff from all professions agreed with this perception of the problem as one of constant crisis – which required constant management.

The second rhetoric utilized by managers was that of neutrality, which was used to present themselves as separate from vested interests and conflicts between the clinical specialties that were a normal feature of hospital organization. The bed managers presented themselves as 'honest brokers' who could act as unbiased arbiters of bed allocation, as this comment from a general manager suggests: 'Somebody has to play heavy honest broker really and say you've got too many beds, you've not got enough, you need to give them to him and so on'.

The third rhetoric was that of rationality, in which the new system was presented as a rational, well-informed alternative to the previous *ad hoc* system, which had clearly not worked. As this quote from a consultant illustrates, the informed, rational basis of the new system was accepted by clinical staff: '[Bed managers] literally know every acute patient – and they've got their finger on the pulse so they know exactly what's going on – they're thinking ahead for the whole week'.

Activity 6.3

1 Would a study like this one be able to evaluate how successful bed management had been in these hospitals?
2 Why do you think the researchers used observation as well as interviews in this study?
3 What sources of bias might affect the findings of this study? How can such sources of bias be reduced?

⟳ **Feedback**

1 In-depth interview data cannot address quantitative questions such as 'How many more patients were admitted in the new system?' They can, however, address questions about process, such as how acceptable the new system was to professionals affected.

2 Observation would provide information about what bed managers did, as well as what they said. It would also provide data about how they interacted with other professionals, as well as their accounts of this interaction.

3 Respondents might want to present their own practice in a positive light, for instance in emphasizing the problems they face (the 'crisis') and their ability to deal with it (the success of bed management). They may tailor their account to what they believe the interviewer wants to hear, so may be influenced by the interviewer's account of the aims of the study. Using other methods (such as observation, examination of hospital records) can help reduce this bias, as can interviewing other professionals. The findings could also be biased as respondents were from only nine hospitals in one city (London) and there is no information about how representative they were. Finally, there is no information here about how the researchers analysed the data, and their selection of illustrative quotes might be biased.

Qualitative interviews, then, unlike participant observation, provide information about what people say rather than what they do. Although this can be a poor guide to what happens in practice, it is useful information in its own right. Language is the main way in which we construct our social world, and examining what, for instance, clinicians and managers say and how they say it provides an account of not only how they perceive the health care system within which they work, but also how they construct it.

As the case study in Activity 6.3 illustrated, researchers might be interested in how people interact in practice, as well as their accounts of interaction with, for example, other health care professionals. In the next chapter you will examine focus group interviews, a method that can address interaction without undertaking a long-term participant observation study.

Summary

Interviews can be more or less structured. Good rapport and thoughtful development of interview topic guides are essential for good data collection. In qualitative work, the interview is used to look at how respondents perceive their world and how their talk helps construct that world.

References

Britten N (1995) Qualitative interviewing in medical research. *British Medical Journal* 311: 251–3.
Cornwell J (1984) *Hard Earned Lives: Accounts of Health and Illness in East London*. London: Tavistock.

Green J and Armstrong D (1993) Controlling the bed state: negotiating hospital organisation. *Sociology of Health and Illness* 15: 337–52.

Green J and Armstrong D (1995) Achieving rational management: bed managers and the crisis in emergency admissions. *The Sociological Review* 43: 744–64.

Sennett R (2003) *Respect: The Formation of Character in an Age of Inequality.* London: Penguin

Further reading

Wengraf T (2001) *Qualitative Research Interviewing.* London: Sage.

Most social science research methods text books have a chapter on interviewing. Two that might be particularly useful as further reading for those doing health research or more applied evaluative research are:

Green J and Thorogood N (2004) In-depth interviews, in Green J and Thorogood N (eds) *Qualitative Methods for Health Research.* London: Sage.

Patton MQ (1990) Qualitative interviewing, in Patton MQ (ed) *Qualitative Evaluation and Research Methods* (2nd edn). Newbury Park, CA: Sage.

Focus groups and other group methods

Judith Green

Overview

Various kinds of group interview have become popular both as methods for collecting data in qualitative studies, and as for involving participants in the research process itself. This chapter introduces you to focus groups and also briefly to some other uses for group processes in health research.

Learning objectives

After working through this chapter, you will be better able to:

- identify the uses and disadvantages of different kinds of group interview as data collection methods
- describe the practical issues to consider in planning a focus group study
- identify how consensus groups can be used in participatory and deliberative projects

Key terms

Deliberative methods Those that enable the participants to develop their own views as part of the process.

Focus groups Groups of people brought together to discuss a topic, with one or more facilitators who introduce and guide the discussion and record it in some way.

Interaction Communication between people.

Natural groups Groups which occur 'naturally', such as workmates or household members.

Group methods

The last chapter considered the one-to-one interview, which has been widely used in health research. One disadvantage of this kind of interview is that it does not provide any access to how people talk to each other in more 'natural' settings. To offset this disadvantage, various kinds of group methods are becoming increasingly popular in both health and health services research. These are used to both collect data from groups of people at the same time, and as a way of involving participants more in the research process.

Jeannine Coreil (1995) makes a useful distinction between four main types of groups that are used in health research (see Table 7.1). In practice, many groups have elements of more than one of these types, but in general, these four headings identify some common aims and processes you might encounter in health research. 'Consensus groups' bring together participants with the explicit aim of coming to a decision about something – perhaps community representatives to identify priorities for health service funding, or clinicians to develop protocols for use in clinical practice. In rural settings, particularly in low-income countries, various kinds of consensus groups have a long history as a way of involving local people in research projects. They are becoming more widely used in high-income countries, with a growing recognition of the usefulness of involving users in policy making and deciding how to implement services. Before describing the main uses of focus groups and natural groups, we will briefly discuss the role of these kinds of consensus groups.

Table 7.1 Coreil's typology of group interviews

Interview type	Features	Typical uses
Consensus group	Often composed of key informants or experts. Aim to develop group consensus. More narrow, closed-ended stimulus material.	Agreeing clinical protocols, resource prioritization.
Focus group	Participants selected to meet sampling criteria. Seeks broad range of ideas of open-ended topic. Formal, controlled pre-arranged time and place. Usually audio-taped and transcribed for analysis.	Testing health promotion materials, exploring service users' views.
Natural group	Group exists independently of the research study. Can be formal or informal (such as an opportunistic interview in the field). Interview guide loosely followed. Recorded by written notes (informal) or audio-taped (formal).	Ethnographic data collection (informal), social research (formal).
Community interview	Open to all or large segments of a community. Usually recorded by written notes.	Project planning, programme evaluation.

(Source: adapted from Coreil 1995)

Consensus groups

There are a number of ways of organizing consensus groups, depending on how much deliberation the group needs and how far the members have to be representative of some wider constituency. Maggie Murphy and colleagues (1998) reviewed consensus methods in the particular context of their uses for developing clinical guidelines. They identify three main types of consensus group. These are:

- *Delphi methods*. In these, the group does not actually meet, but the members all complete a questionnaire on their views on a particular topic. Examples might be priorities for research in a certain area, or the most important elements to include on a new training curriculum. In stage 2, participants receive a collated summary of all responses. They are then asked to revise judgements in the light of these responses from others in the group. This cycle might be repeated until a group consensus or summary of differing views can be reported.
- *Nominal group techniques*. These are ways of formalizing group decision making such that all members contribute, and have an opportunity to deliberate on their views. This is a useful method for coming up with priorities for action. The basic process involves each participant first individually noting their own ideas. These are then all listed in a group setting, discussed by the group, then voted on. Votes are statistically analysed to identify strength of agreement and disagreement.
- *Consensus development conference*. This usually involves an open meeting, at which the participants discuss the topic, but also hear evidence from experts in order to deliberate on areas of agreement, rather like a jury in a legal trial. Murphy *et al.* (1998) identified a number of topics in the health field in which consensus conferences had been used, including treatment of stroke, the management of hypertension and the diagnosis of depression in later life.

Delphi groups, nominal group techniques and consensus development conferences are typically used with professionals as formal methods for collecting expert opinion when there is insufficient other evidence on which to base policy. However, community members are also experts in their own health, and on the services that their communities need. Citizens' juries have become popular as a way of involving communities in decisions about, for instance, the management of environmental hazards, or the development of guidelines for managing health problems. Similar to consensus development conferences, these are facilitated meetings that involve deliberations in which the participants hear evidence from various experts during the decision-making process. Group techniques that aim to allow participants to come to some informed decisions are often called deliberative group processes. Although the aim is usually policy development (for instance, to include users' views in the shaping of policy implementation) they are also used to produce research data. Such techniques are especially useful when the researcher wants access to how decisions are made.

Focus groups and natural groups

Focus groups consist of a number (typically from eight to 12, although this depends on the aim of the study) of people brought together to discuss a topic, with one or more facilitators who introduce and guide the discussion and record it in some way. Sometimes the group is also asked to carry out exercises together, such as sorting cards with statements on them, or ranking a list of priorities. Focus groups provide an opportunity to research not only people's experiences and attitudes, but how these are communicated in a relatively 'naturalistic' setting. In community development projects they are also a research technique that can help to involve a community with the research process. For instance, carrying out a focus group study before introducing a vaccination programme for villages in a rural area not only informs the researchers about the villagers' attitudes to vaccination but also potentially informs the villagers about the research programme. If the results from focus groups do inform the research, then a community may be more committed to the results of that research.

✐ Activity 7.1

What advantages might focus groups have over participant observation?

↻ Feedback

They are a more efficient method of collecting data on a topic, as the facilitator can set the agenda and prompt for particular areas to be discussed in more depth. They are also potentially less intrusive than participant observation.

Choice of participants is important. The sample does not usually represent the larger population in any statistical way but may be chosen to reflect the range of people in whom the researcher is interested. Traditionally, focus groups were used in market research where participants did not know each other before the group met. In health research, researchers often sample *peer groups*, or participants who already know each other or at least have something in common. Natural groups are a particular kind of focus group in which the participants already know each other, perhaps as work colleagues, friends or those from the same social club. This could be groups of nurses who work on the same ward, patients who run a self-help group, or people who live together in the same household. There is a wide range of possible uses for focus group methods, including using them to test research instruments (such as questionnaires) to observe how the language used in the questions is understood by different groups in the population. In developing health care interventions, such as health education campaigns, focus groups can be used to see how messages are received, understood and communicated to others.

M. Khan and Lenore Manderson (1992) suggest that, in practice, many interviews in developing country settings will be informal 'natural' group interviews. As researchers start asking questions, more people will join in, and a group interview happens spontaneously. The everyday demands of people coming and going or work being done often interrupt attempts at more structured interview formats. As they note, this can be a real bonus as:

> Such natural clusterings of people represent, in a loose fashion, the resources upon which any member of the group might draw . . . This is a group that may

weave or mend nets together . . . It is precisely this natural social network which provides the scripting for the management of an illness event – what to do with a child with bloody diarrhoea, for example . . . Decisions about such matters are rarely carried out by one care-giver alone: people draw on those around them. As a result, discussions with such groups provide fairly accurate data regarding the diagnosis and treatment of illness, choices of health services, and so on.

Thus natural groups are an invaluable resource for accessing not only what kind of health knowledge a community has but how that knowledge is transmitted to others, discussed in everyday contexts and acted upon. In more formal settings than those described by Khan and Manderson, natural groups can be brought together in a research setting with the aim of recreating (to some extent) the kinds of everyday discussions that might occur around health topics. Jenny Kitzinger (1994) used such groups in a study of how media messages about HIV/AIDS were understood by various audiences in a UK context. She notes that in the study:

> We chose to work with pre-existing groups – clusters of people who already knew each other through living, working or socialising together. We did this is order to explore how people might talk about AIDS within the various and overlapping groupings within which they actually operate. Flatmates, colleagues and friends – these are precisely the people with whom one might 'naturally' discuss such topics . . . The fact that research participants already knew each other had the additional advantage that [they] could relate each other's comments to actual incidents in their daily shared lives. They often challenged each other on contradictions between what they were professing to believe and how they actually behaved.

Thus Kitzinger is also suggesting that group discussion can provide some access to what people do, as well as what they say they do. Again, this is a potential advantage compared with interviews. However, it should be remembered that a focus group – even if the participants know each other already – is still not a 'natural' setting. Few groups of friends will gather to discuss one topic for a hour or two, and what they say to a moderator may well not reflect what they might say if no researchers were present.

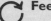 **Activity 7.2**

What do focus groups provide that one-to-one interviews can't?

Feedback

Focus groups provide access to *how* participants interact with each other. This can be useful because the researcher can see how opinions are received by others – whether they are challenged or agreed with, for instance. The relatively informal group setting can also encourage talk about topics that might be sensitive, such as sexual behaviour. However, groups may be inhibiting for some participants, who may feel unable to give their opinions, particularly if they are likely to be marginal to those of the rest of the group.

In many health care systems, focus groups can be a good way to access patient attitudes to health care services, or staff attitudes to quality standards. They can also be used to inform resource allocation by, for instance, asking groups from the population about priorities for health care spending.

Adapting methods for the setting

Bilkis Vissandjée, Shelly Abdool and Sophie Dupéré (2002) discuss the need to adapt the methods used to the particular setting you are working in. Drawing on their experiences of running focus groups in rural India for a project on the influence of rural women's autonomy on their health, they make some suggestions for designing what they call 'culturally competent' focus groups:

- Detailed and careful planning and implementation, so that participants know what to expect from the research (and, as importantly, what not to expect) and to build relationships. This must be done in collaboration with those who know the setting well.
- Consider the daily lives of participants – what timing and location will fit best for the men and women you would like to talk to? In rural India, it was important to find locations in which women could talk without being overheard.
- How will you deal with onlookers? In many settings, it would be typical for all villagers to be asked to a social occasion, so inviting only some may well mean that others gather to watch.
- Consider local hierarchies, and how they will affect both how willing all participants are to speak and what can be said. In rural India, the researchers had to consider age, gender, caste, religion and family position (such as daughter-in-law relative to mother-in-law). Although they could hold separate focus groups for men and women, it was not possible to separate groups by caste. This meant that those women who were of lower caste or education often did not speak in the groups. Similarly, daughters-in-law had less autonomy to speak in meetings than their mothers-in-law.
- Ethics. Written assurances of confidentiality and written consent forms would be negatively viewed in this context, as associated with government affairs. The researchers thus had to use verbal explanations and assurances. Another ethical issue to consider when discussing sensitive topics in rural settings is that of 'over-disclosure'. Participants should not be encouraged to disclose information that could be difficult to manage in future everyday contexts.
- Follow up. In this research, women might feel that the focus group discussion raised difficult issues for them, or led them to question taken-for-granted ways of life. It was important to follow up with oral interviews to give women a chance to reflect on the group discussion.

In conclusion, Vissandjée, Abdool and Dupéré (2002) suggest that developing appropriate methods for the setting requires detailed ethnographic work as a prerequisite, and a good understanding of local social, cultural and political contexts.

✏ Activity 7.3

1   Can you think of some research topics that might be particularly suitable for focus group interviews?
2   Are there any kinds of research for which you would avoid using focus groups?

↻ Feedback

1   Your ideas will be informed by your knowledge of topics likely to generate group discussion. In most cultures, there are some topics on which respondents have a 'story' to tell: for example, about experience of childbirth, or of visiting a general practitioner.

These stories are often told more readily (and differently) in group settings than in one-to-one interviews.

2   Again, the answer to this will depend on social context. Every culture has areas of behaviour that are seen as 'private' and may be unsuitable for group discussions. Political constraints might also limit the use of focus groups. In a hierarchical work setting (such as most hospital departments), including workers from all grades might inhibit some in giving their opinions.

Running focus groups

The key to successful focus groups is careful preparation. We've already suggested that this involves thinking about appropriate methods for the cultural setting, thinking about what kind of data you need, and who will provide it, whether natural groups, if you want to maximize interaction between participants, or perhaps a more heterogeneous group if you want a broad range of opinions within each group. Sampling appropriately usually means some kind of purposive sampling, in which you think about which participants and groups of participants will best generate data to answer your research question. Some possibilities for recruitment include:

- Advertising for volunteers, for instance on community notice boards, through email lists or in hospital waiting rooms. This is fine for some pilot studies, or for accessing participants who might be hard to reach, although often response rates are very low.
- Working with established community groups to recruit volunteers, such as schools, voluntary organizations or patients' associations.
- Using existing sampling frames (lists of medical professionals, addresses from electoral rolls) to invite people to participate. Care must be taken that it is legal and ethical to use lists in this way.

Some of the issues you need to consider in planning a focus group study are: the topic guide, facilitation, location and resources.

The topic guide

A focus group topic guide is similar to a topic guide for semi-structured interviews (see Chapter 6) in that it should list the topics you want to cover, and some prompts that will stimulate discussion. Here are some suggested tips for developing focus group topic guides.

The introduction is a brief summary of the aims of the group, how long it will take, what will happen to the data and assurances of confidentiality.

Start with 'ice-breaker' exercises to ensure everyone speaks and gets to know each other a little. These should include the participants' identifying themselves by the name they like to use.

You might want to follow up with a *focusing exercise* designed to get participants thinking about the topic. This might, for instance, ask participants to rank words or pictures in order of importance

Start with *general questions* about the topic. Move on to more *specific questions*, but do not include more than about five key questions. These might include:

Questions on experiences. (What happened? What did you do?)
Questions on attitudes to experiences. (How did you feel about that?)
Questions on what participants like/dislike about services.
Questions about what could be improved now/in an ideal world.

Avoid asking questions starting 'Why . . .?' These are ambiguous, and can often sound interrogative. Make sure questions are *simple*, easy to understand, and open ended. Pilot them first with colleagues.

Think about some *prompts and probes* to get the group to expand on these and to broaden discussion if one person is dominating. These might include:

Has anyone else had this experience?
What else do you like/dislike?
OK, thanks for that contribution. Do other people feel as strongly?

Summing up. Finish by summarizing the key points raised in the discussion. Ask if anything has been missed or if participants want to add anything. Thank participants for attending and hand out any travel expenses or incentives.

The topic guide should be piloted to ensure that the questions and instructions for tasks are understood by participants and work well to generate discussion.

Facilitation

Focus groups are usually facilitated by one person (often called the moderator) assisted by one other person or more to record discussion and/or make sure tape recorders are running, help with meeting and greeting and organizing refreshments. Moderators need skills in running discussions and making participants feel respected and listened to. Often, they need some knowledge of the topic area as well. For some groups you will need particular skills or attributes, such as competence in local languages, or perhaps social attributes or experiences that match those of the participants.

Location

Choosing an appropriate venue and time is essential. This should be somewhere all participants will feel comfortable in. Often a room in a community centre or local school is more familiar than a hospital location or university seminar room. Make sure there is a quiet enough room in which to hold the discussion, and that the location is one all participants can get to and into easily. Consider whether you will also need to provide childcare facilities, or transport. Set out furniture so that there are no physical barriers to interaction: a circle of chairs usually works best. In cultures where it is the norm for people to bring others, consider how you will accommodate them: do you need a separate room for these 'extras' or will you be able to fit them into the group discussion?

Resources

It is usual to offer refreshments, depending on local norms. A meal can be a good incentive for people to volunteer for the group. You may also want to consider financial incentives. In high-income countries, market research companies usually pay participants, and many focus group volunteers may now expect to be paid for their time. However, in other settings this could be insensitive or divisive and may be seen as unethical. Other incentives may be preferable, such as store vouchers or gifts.

Resources for running the group will include recording equipment and tapes, perhaps flip charts for writing up key points and summaries, any materials you need for the ice breaking and other exercises and travel expenses for the participants.

Activity 7.4

You have been asked to organize some focus groups to explore how mothers prevent accidents to their children. The women have been recruited from primary care centres and do not know each other.

1 Think of one appropriate ice-breaking and one appropriate focusing exercise for your groups.
2 Think of three or four questions for a topic guide that would generate discussion on this issue.

Feedback

1 One possibility is to ask each participant to introduce themselves by saying their name, and one kind of food they like, and one they don't like. Or two facts about themselves: one true, and the other a lie. The key is to think of questions that people will not be embarrassed to answer, and will not generate discomfort: this is clearly dependant on the participants and the cultural setting. A focusing exercise might get the group to look at pictures of playgrounds, kitchens and outdoor environments to rank

them in order of how likely children are to have accidents there, or to identify the main risks of injury to children.

2 Some suggestions might be:

'Has anyone's child had an accident recently?' 'Anyone else?'
'What happened? How did it happen?
'What did you do?'
'What do you do in the house/while out to prevent accidents?'

If possible, try out your exercises and questions with mothers of young children. Do they work?

Focus groups for needs assessment

In many health care systems there are policy initiatives that encourage those who provide or commission health care services to seek the views of users on their perceived needs for health care and their attitudes to services currently offered. Focus groups have been increasingly used to assist in this kind of needs assessment. In the next activity, there are some extracts from a British report to the National Health Service Executive, which is an example of this kind of use of focus group methods. Read the following extract by Allsop and colleagues (1995)

South Asians with Diabetes: Their Experiences of Primary Care and the Relevance of Current Satisfaction Methods:

The incidence of diabetes is significantly higher in the British south Asian communities than in the British population as a whole. It has also been shown that there is a high proportion of undiagnosed cases in these communities. [One aim of] this research was to obtain indicative views from south Asians with diabetes about their experiences of care and their satisfaction and dissatisfaction with the provision they had received . . . We collected and analysed three types of data: data from short questionnaires, focus groups, and notes from meetings with community coordinators and interpreters. Focus group participants were recruited by community workers.

[Focus group] discussion was based on a *questioning route* which is a logical sequence of open-ended questions which encourage universal participation within the group . . . The themes we included in the questioning route began with each individual's personal history of diabetes following their own illness pathway. The themes were when, and how, people were diagnosed and their reactions to their diagnosis. This was followed by a section asking about their contact with health care professionals . . . Two focus groups met in each of three inner-city sites. Overall, the focus groups included members of the main ethnic groups which make up the south Asian population in Britain.

Groups were single sex on two sites, where local custom required segregation of the sexes. The dominant attitude in all groups was one of acceptance of the diagnosis of diabetes and indeed good humour. There was also a degree of fatalism. The overwhelming impression was that while a minority were well controlled [in managing their diabetes] and understood their condition, many were not. [Problems were reported] in relation to the ease of communication with health care professionals and access to information and advice in their own language and within the context of their own customs and practices. This resulted in most participants lacking adequate information, advice and support . . .

Because of their reluctance to voice dissatisfaction, many of the participants' concerns were implicit. Directly expressed dissatisfaction included concerns about the numbers of different doctors seen in hospital settings, long waiting times in clinics, conflicting advice given by various people involved in their care, receptionists who acted inappropriately as interpreters. Implicitly expressed dissatisfaction included concerns about health problems not being addressed, absence of information on diet in a form people could understand, and lack of low-cost facilities for taking exercise.

Activity 7.5

1 Suggest some reasons why focus groups may have been chosen for this study.
2 How did the researchers try to ensure that all members of the groups could contribute?
3 What are the possible limitations of this kind of data?

Feedback

1 There is a suggestion that access to health care may be limited (as diabetes may be under-diagnosed), so discussions may raise some reasons for this. South Asians in Britain, although from a range of different backgrounds, may share common problems in dealing with a health service which is not responsive to their needs, and focus groups allow participants to draw on shared experience. Given that patients are often reluctant to criticize health services, the informal approach of the focus group may be a more effective way of uncovering dissatisfaction.

2 They used a 'questioning route' to canvass experiences from all members in the groups. They also held single-sex groups when this was appropriate.

3 The three sites are unlikely to be representative of the whole south Asian population, even if the participants were similar in terms of ethnicity. As the members were recruited by community coordinators, the groups themselves might not be representative. It would be difficult to gauge the views of undiagnosed diabetics. Data from focus groups, like those from qualitative interviews and participant observation, can be difficult to organize and analyse for novice researchers. If the discussion is audio- or videotaped and transcribed, an enormous amount of data can be collected. The task of analysing these data is the subject of the next chapter.

Summary

Group interviews are a useful method for generating data about how social knowledge is constructed and can be particularly suitable for participatory research. They have an advantage over participant observation in that they are relatively efficient, and an advantage over one-to-one interviews in that they provide access to interaction. The disadvantages are that they can take considerable time and effort to set up. Groups need skilled moderators, recruitment can be slow and data can be difficult and time-consuming to analyse.

References

Allsop J, Tritter J, Turner G and Elliot B (1995) *South Asians with Diabetes: Their Experiences of Primary Care and the Relevance of Current Satisfaction Methods.* London: Social Science Research Centre, South Bank University.

Coreil J (1995) Group interview methods in community health research. *Medical Anthropology* 16: 193–210.

Khan ME and Manderson L (1992) Focus groups in tropical diseases research. *Health Policy and Planning* 7: 56–66.

Kitzinger J (1994) The methodology of focus groups: the importance of interaction between research participants. *Sociology of Health and Illness* 16: 103–21.

Murphy MK, Black NA, Lamping DL, McKee CM, Sanderson CFB, Askham J, Marteau T (1998) Consensus development methods, and their use in clinical guideline development. *Health Technology Assessment* 2 (3): 1–88.

Vissandjée B, Abdool S and Dupéré S (2002) Focus groups in rural Gujarat, India: a modified approach. *Qualitative Health Research* 12: 826–43.

Further reading

Krueger R and Casey MA (2000) *Focus Groups: A Practical Guide for Applied Research* (3rd edn). Thousand Oaks, CA: Sage.

A useful guidebook full of practical advice on the whole process of focus group research, from planning, recruiting, and running groups through to analysing and reporting the data generated. The authors draw from their own experiences of running different kinds of focus groups, largely in North America.

Barbour R and Kitzinger J (eds) (1999) *Developing Focus Group Research: Politics, Theory and Practice.* London: Sage.

A collection of chapters drawing on authors' empirical experiences of focus group research that cover methodological issues including the impact of context, using focus groups in feminist and participatory research, using focus groups for sensitive topics and approaches to analysis. This collection gives a good flavour of the range of uses, advantages and limitations of various kinds of group interviews.

8 Analysing qualitative data
Judith Green

Overview

This chapter describes the basics of thematic analysis of qualitative data, introduces some approaches for more sophisticated analysis and suggests some ways of improving the quality of qualitative analysis.

Learning objectives

After working through this chapter, you will be better able to:

- identify the main objectives of qualitative analysis
- undertake a basic thematic analysis of qualitative data
- understand how reliability and validity can be maximized in qualitative research

Key terms

Coding The process by which data extracts are labelled as indicators of a concept.

Introduction

To illustrate some of the principles of qualitative analysis, this chapter draws on some examples of data from a small qualitative study carried out in the UK of bilingual young people's accounts of interpreting in health care settings (Free *et al.* 2003). Here is a summary of the study.

The bilingual young people's study

In London, many GPs report that they are often asked to consult with patients who do not speak English and who bring their children to the consultation to help interpret. This raises a number of problems. First, children may not have sufficient language skills to interpret accurately. Second, GPs feel that for many health care problems children are inappropriate interpreters, either because they will have to translate personal information for their parents or they will lack general knowledge about health and illness. Third, having to help their families may mean that children miss school or college. There was already a large literature on these problems and how they could be addressed by improving the professional interpreting services on offer. However, there was no literature on what young people thought about their contribution. This study was carried out to find out what the young interpreters themselves felt about their experiences: why they helped their families, what they liked and didn't like about this work and what suggestions could be made to improve their families' access to health care. Interviews were held with 77 young people aged between nine and 18 who spoke English and at least one other language and who had some experience of interpreting for others. The findings from this study suggested why young interpreters are sometimes used by preference, and also had some implications for GPs.

Approaches to analysing qualitative data

One of the most difficult stages of research for the novice qualitative researcher is that of analysis: what to do with the data (field notes or transcripts of interviews) that are produced. This section introduces some of the principles of coding and analysing data from interviews, focus groups, or field notes from participant observation studies. There are a number of different ways of approaching analysis, depending on your theoretical orientation, disciplinary background and the aims of the study, but there are several objectives many of these approaches share. These are as follows.

Describing the form and nature of phenomena and developing conceptual definitions

In Chapters 1 and 5 you learnt about the idea that qualitative research aims to explore the meaning of phenomena. Analysis is often, then, directed at developing in-depth descriptions of phenomena that reflect the complexity of social life and the development of conceptual definitions that contribute to further research.

Describing typologies and classifications

As well as representing the complexity of your data, analysis also has to represent the major findings or key themes for the reader. Typologies are one way of doing this. If you look back at Chapter 5, you will see how the researchers described a typology of responses to asthma diagnosis: 'deniers', 'acceptors' and 'pragmatists'. These typologies are drawn up by looking for patterns in how people give accounts of their health and illness, or health-seeking behaviour. Note that they are derived from the data, not from looking for comparisons between pre-existing variables such as gender or age. As well looking at the content of what is said, it is sometimes helpful to examine how people talk about things. For example, one typology developed in the bilingual young people's study was that of 'straightforward' and 'problematic' consultations. There was a key difference between how these were described in the interviews, with 'straightforward' consultations being described in very brief accounts of the encounter (such as 'I just explained to my mum what the doctor said, and that was that') whereas 'problematic' encounters were often told as longer and more elaborated stories.

Identifying associations between attitudes, behaviours and experiences

Qualitative research does not aim to find statistical associations, but nevertheless explores connections within the data through comparing patterns in accounts of attitudes, behaviours and experiences. In the study of asthma patients you looked at in Chapter 5, these included associations between patients' attitudes to their diagnosis (denial, acceptance or pragmatism) and their behaviour – in this case their use of medication (using reliever medication only, using medications exactly as prescribed by the doctor or adapting the doctor's advice).

New ideas and theories

Although health research is often orientated towards practical outcomes and may be addressing a tight research question, ideally new ideas and theories will also emerge from the data. Some of these will be useful for sensitizing practitioners or policy makers to issues they may not have thought about, or different ways of looking at some aspect of health. Some may not have immediate relevance to the provision of better health care but they may feed into a broader understanding of the context in which health care happens, or may help us think differently about some taken-for-granted aspect of practice. For instance, in the bilingual young people's study, one outcome of the analysis was a reconceptualization of young people's contribution as 'work' rather than as 'poor interpreting'. Thinking about their contribution as 'work' enables us to think differently about it: rather than assuming that it is just a 'problem', and asking how we can remove the need for it, we can ask in what circumstances is it easier or harder to do? Is it ever financially remunerated and what difference does this make to how they experience it?

First steps in analysis

Whatever the aims of analysis, there are some common 'first steps' in organizing and preparing data.

Begin analysis at the beginning of the project

This is essential for qualitative analysis. In quantitative studies, analysis is usually a separate stage after data collection. In qualitative research, analysis should begin as soon as you start collecting data. This is in part to maximize the flexibility of qualitative designs. As you begin analysing, new theories emerge to test, suggesting new data to collect or refinements of the interview topic guide.

Preparing your data

Interview transcripts should be laid out with enough space to write notes and codes on the manuscript. It is helpful to number both pages and lines for ease of reference. In Table 8.1 we have reproduced an extract from a transcript from the

30   **A** My Dad he has no problems understanding or speaking
31   English, he is alright about that, but, umm basically when   } OBLIGATION/DUTY
32   we go to doctor and things like that, one of us has to go   TO HELP
33   with my Mum

34   **Int** yeah

35   **A** You know, she can't explain certain things and you
36   know, especially with the family doctor now that we change } STRATEGIES to manage
37   to a Bengali doctor, that's fine with her but before she   (FIRST LANGUAGE GP)
38   used to have a lot of problems, you know, like explain and   }
39   things that, even making a phone call, emergency phone call } PROBLEMS (EMERGENCIES)
40   or things like that she couldn't, because when you are at   \   (PHONE ACCESS)
41   school or at college or things like that and when she has   } DISADVANTAGES OF CHILDREN
42   some problems she couldn't speak to anyone so that's why we } STRATEGIES to manage
43   had to change to a Bengali doctor for her   /   (FIRST LANGUAGE GP)
...
52   ..... but when we go to hospital, they do ask you   } STRATEGIES to manage
54   like, do you need interpreters and things like that -   /   (USE OF FORMAL SERVICES)

55   **Int** - yes -

56   **A** - on the form, you know to send it back so they will   SHARED RESPONSIBILITY
57   arrange someone for you but we don't do that basically,
58   cause we go with her cause its easier for her, for her to   } REASONS FOR USING CHILDREN
59   explain to us than to the other person, 'cause they don't | (PERSONAL KNOWLEDGE)
60   know what they, how they are going to translate and things |
61   like that, and we know about her, how she is feeling and |
62   things like that so we could translate easier for her   ___ UNPROBLEMATIC TRANSLATION
...
81   **Int** You said that before when your Mum used to be with a
82   doctor that wasn't Bangladeshi ....
83   can you sort of tell me about the kinds of problems she had?

89   **A** I mean, she couldn't explain what her problem is, you ⌐] DISRUPTED COMMUNICATION
90   know and although we were more young that time   ⌐   (INTERPRETER'S SKILLS)
91   and if she explained something to us, we couldn't | (PATIENT'S SKILLS)
92   translate it the way she wanted ... |

118   ... but before I was about   ⌐ DISRUPTED COMMUNICATION
120   12, 13 when I used to go with my Mum so that was really | (LACK of SOPHISTICATION)
121   hard for me basically   ⌐
123   I used to find it really difficult to explain it for her
124   ... I don't know, 'cause there is certain problems she has ⌐ DISRUPTED COMMUNICATION
127   that I have, I don't have any experience about   ⌐   (LACK of EXPERIENCE)
129   you know, sort of personal problems and things like ⌐
130   that, I don't know what was she talking about so I just/ DISRUPTED COMMUNICATION
                                                                      (LACK of EXPERIENCE)
                                                                    + inappropriate for
                                                                       age?

Table 8.1 Extract from coded interview transcript.
This is an interview with a young woman, bilingual and English, discussing her experiences of
interpreting for her family. The interviewer's talk is marked (Int) and the interviewee is A.

Source: Free et al 2003

bilingual young people's study to illustrate what a transcript looks like after initial coding, although you may find it easier to double space the lines. Field notes and interview notes should be typed up as soon as possible after collection. If you have assured participants of confidentiality, make sure transcripts or field notes do not contain names, only identifiers that are linked with names on a separate record, which should be kept securely.

Organizing the data

Your data must be organized so that you can find extracts easily, refer back to the original source when necessary and keep a record of what has been done. In a large project, it soon becomes difficult to keep track of notes, tapes and transcripts unless you have a good system for labelling and filing them. A number of software packages now exist that are designed to help organize and manage qualitative data. These are briefly discussed below. If you are using one of these, you may need to check the requirements before preparing the data for analysis.

Familiarizing yourself with the data

You need to be familiar with your own data. Read and re-read notes and transcripts, listen to tape recordings and familiarize yourself with the content and format of the data. Write summaries of each interview, or period in the field, if this helps.

Thematic analysis

Many approaches to qualitative analysis rely on identifying key themes, or recurring issues, in the data. In many health studies, this is the main aim of analysis: to identify those issues that commonly emerge in interviews or focus groups, or that emerge as general headings under which we can describe most of the data. To identify key themes, we need to look closely at the data to see patterns. This first involves beginning to code the data, a process that has three overlapping stages.

Initial coding

Each transcript, or set of notes, is read in detail, with the analyst making notes in the margin on 'what is going on here': what is the participant referring to, or talking about. As you can see in Table 8.1, initial coding of this section of transcript has identified a number of issues in this young woman's accounts of her experience, including *strategies to manage* health care interactions when parents don't speak English, causes of *disrupted communication* and accounts of *unproblematic translation* experiences.

Developing a coding scheme

These margin notes are collated and discussed by the project team. They are then sorted into categories and subcategories: this is the coding scheme. For instance, if you look at the codes written on the margin of the transcript in Table 8.1, some of them refer to 'Disrupted communication'. This was a major category in this study, which was broken down into a number of subcategories to cover the various causes to which participants attributed disruptions in communication in medical settings:

1) Causes of disrupted communication:
    a) Communication skills of patient (vocabulary/other)
    b) Communication skills of interpreter (vocabulary/other)
    c) Communication skills of professionals (vocabulary/other)
    d) Experience of interpreter
    e) etc . . .

Each of these codes should be named and perhaps a brief description added to define it. It is also helpful to keep notes about any emerging ideas about the data as you go through this process. At this stage, it is important to discuss your coding scheme, and get other people to help code if possible. This will minimize the chance of you missing important issues, or being funnelled into narrow interpretations.

✐ Activity 8.1

The transcript in Table 8.1 has been annotated by one researcher, in the context of a project with specific aims. However, there are many other potential themes here. Look at the data as if you were interested in the topics of roles within the family in terms of accessing health care. Are there any lines that you might code for this theme, and what might you call your code?

↻ Feedback

Lines 30 to 33 discuss the difference between the interviewee's mother and father in terms of need for interpreting. You might want to provisionally code these 'Parents' needs for interpreting'. In lines 118 to 120, she discusses her role when younger: this might be 'Young children's roles'. Lines 61 to 62 refer to the interviewee's accounts of why family members might help (their 'knowing how she is feeling'): this might be something like 'Emotional work'. You may well have come up with different examples or codes. There are no 'right' or 'wrong' codes, only coding schemes that will work more or less well at helping you see what is in the data and what associations there are within them.

Coding the data

New data are then coded as they are added to the data set. New cases will challenge emerging coding schemes, which need to be flexible enough to be adapted as you rethink categories and subcategories.

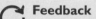 **Activity 8.2**

Here is a short extract from another transcript from the bilingual children's study:

Interviewer: So tell me more about that visit [to the doctor] for your mum's medicine? Why was that one difficult?

Young man: Well, she was telling my mum why she had to have this new medicine, and I was telling my mum, and she understood, but like she didn't want to take the pills, she was happy with the ones she had already, so I'm like telling the doctor 'my mum doesn't want to change to these pills' but like the doctor thinks I haven't explained properly, so she keeps like saying 'tell her again' and it was like, but I can't convince my mum – that's her decision whether she wants the new pills or not.

How might you code this extract?

Feedback

You may have put this under a new subcategory of causes of disrupted communication, such as 'Conflicts between doctor and patient', or you might have decided that this was a new category, such as 'Conflicts between the roles of interpreter and advocate'. If the category 'Causes of disruption' becomes too large, it might be sensible to split this up and think about the subcategories in more detail.

'Cut and paste'

Once some of the data are coded we can continue exploring the data using 'cut-and-paste' techniques in which the coded extracts from a number of cases are collected under the same headings. This can be done manually, by literally cutting up copies of transcripts and then pasting them onto large sheets of paper, or sorting them into piles, each with a code heading. With small data sets, this can be very effective, and you (and the rest of the team) can see how the data are sorted, and move extracts around. Use different coloured paper, or different fonts, on each transcript so you can refer back to see where each extract came from. An alternative is to use a word processor to electronically 'cut and paste' extracts to a set of files, one for each category (or subcategory) in the coding scheme.

As you start collecting extracts under each heading, they can be compared with each other, and more themes start emerging. You will probably want to revisit your coding scheme to split some categories, or combine others, or rethink completely what some are 'about'.

These kinds of cut-and-paste techniques are 'low technology' but they work. They allow the researcher, or team of researchers, to compare, contrast, start to build up categories and typologies and to discuss the 'meaning' of their data. With larger data sets you may have to type in a case identifier for the original transcript after each quote. At this point, the advantages of using computer software to help with the analysis start emerging (see below).

The key headings from your coding scheme can be the basis for sections of your report. For instance, one report from the bilingual young people's project used the following headings, which were derived from three main categories in the coding scheme: experiences of interpreting, accounts of 'straightforward' interpreting and disrupted communication (Free *et al.* 2003).

Developing more intensive qualitative analysis

Often a thematic analysis is appropriate to the study aims. Sometimes, though, if the data are rich enough, we might want to carry out a more thorough analysis and develop a more sophisticated understanding of the data. Two particular approaches to qualitative analysis have become popular in the field of health research: framework analysis and grounded theory. This section does not aim to show you how to do analysis using these methods, but to introduce the main principles so you can judge research reports that claim to have used them.

Framework analysis

This is an approach developed specifically for more applied qualitative research, so it has an appeal to many of those working in public health and related fields. It was developed by researchers at what is now the UK National Centre for Social Research (http://www.scpr.ac.uk) and described by Jane Ritchie and Liz Spencer (1994) as:

> an analytical process which involves a number of distinct, though highly interconnected, stages . . . although systematic and disciplined, it relies on the creative and conceptual ability of the analyst to determine meaning, salience and connections . . . The strength of an approach like 'Framework' is that by following a well-defined procedure, it is possible to reconsider and rework ideas precisely because the analytical process has been documented and is therefore accessible.

Framework analysis is particularly appropriate when the study is tightly orientated towards policy outcomes and has clear aims at the outset. Ritchie and Spencer describe five stages in framework analysis. These are:

- *Familiarization.* To get a feel for the whole data set, its range and diversity, and perhaps (if only using a sample of the data for the report) selecting a representative sample for full analysis.
- *Identifying a thematic framework.* This is like the process of developing a coding scheme in the thematic approach. For framework analysis, though, these key themes are likely to reflect the aims of the original proposal as well as those emerging from the data. The headings might, then, reflect the original questions in the topic guide, although it is important to be inductive as well. This is then

developed into an index, which lists all the categories to be used in the analysis. It is helpful to number these.

- *Indexing.* The thematic framework is then applied to the whole data set. The number relating to the sub-category in the index is written in the margin of the transcript.
- *Charting.* Charting has the same function as 'cut and paste', in that data are then rearranged according to appropriate thematic references in charts, so that themes can be compared across cases. Table 8.2 is an example of what such charts may look like, using data from the bilingual young people's study. Note that summaries of data can be used as well as direct quotes, but there is still a reference to the original source.
- *Mapping and interpretation.* These charts, and any notes made while developing the thematic framework, are then reviewed to look at patterns across the data and associations within it. This process involves defining concepts, mapping the range and nature of phenomena, creating typologies and making provisional explanations of associations within the data. For example, in the bilingual young people's study, some key patterns and associations were around the settings in which interpreted communication was most likely to be successful or unsuccessful. We therefore looked for associations between contexts and reported problems, and the kinds of health care issues being described and whether communication was successful or not.

Finally, as this kind of analysis is policy orientated, an important element is identifying strategies for improving health care. These can be either those identified directly by participants, or those that can be inferred from the kinds of problems they describe facing. Thus, in the bilingual young people's study, several young people talked about the difficulty of interpreting when professionals did not look at them, only at the client. Here is one example of a comment about this, from a 14-year old:

> When I'm with my Mum at the doctor's, what's really difficult is that the doctors sometime just look at my Mum, not me, even if it's me that's doing the talking. I find that really hard, 'cause I don't know if the doctor is hearing me, or what. I expect that if you're talking to a person, they look you in the face, so you can communicate properly. I hate it when they just ignore me.

 Activity 8.3

Look at the extract above. How might you use this in making some policy suggestions in a report on this data?

Feedback

Looking at the client, not the interpreter, is of course 'good practice' if working with a professional interpreter, but young people often found it very disruptive. One possible policy suggestion might be to amend advice given to health professionals when working with young informal interpreters, to look at them as well as the client.

Table 8.2 Sections of possible charts from the bilingual young people's study

1. Disrupters of good communication – Bengali speakers

Number	Age, gender	Summary of experiences	Problematic encounters	Sources of disruption 1 – own language skills	Sources of disruption 2 – parents' behaviour
B1	13, F	Accompanies mum to doctors etc., interprets for officials, translates letters to house.	Council officer (p. 6). Dentist (p. 10).	'Don't know words' (p. 5).	'Mum interrupts when I'm on phone' (p. 6).
B2	15, F	Helps for past year, now older sister has left home – phoning GP, accompanies mum to parents evenings.	None – all 'no problems' (p. 3).	N/A	N/A
B9	14, M	Interprets for mum and grandmother (hospital, GP, dentist).	One visit abandoned ('woman's problem') (p. 7), dentist (p. 11).	Didn't know Bengali words (p. 12).	Sometimes parents/grand-mother argue with you while you're trying to translate (p. 13).

2. Disrupters of communication – Albanian speakers

Number	Age, gender	Summary of experiences	Problematic encounters	Sources of disruption 1 – own language skills	Sources of disruption 2 – parents' behaviour
A1	16, M	Helps friends (solicitor), helped stranger register with GP.	Registering with GP (p. 7).	'English not good when I came' (p. 4).	N/A
A2	15, F	Helps 'others in community'.	Social services (p. 9).	Sometimes don't know English words (p. 6).	N/A
A10	14, M				

Source: Free et al 2003

Grounded theory

This approach, also called the 'constant comparative method' is a more inductive approach than framework analysis, in that it aims to stay grounded in the empirical data rather than in the original aims of the study. This means that the research question, sampling strategy, sample, and key outputs of the study can be very different from those originally identified. For this reason, it is perhaps less suited to more applied health research, where tight timescales and the need for defined outputs for commissioners mean there can be less flexibility in research design. However, the techniques of grounded theory have been widely used in many social research projects, and many researchers utilize a 'grounded theory' approach to some extent in their analysis.

Grounded theory is associated with two North American sociologists, Barney Glaser and Anselm Strauss (Strauss 1987), who believed that the process of qualitative analysis could be 'demystified' by developing some rules of thumb for what they called 'the discovery of theory from data'. As this term suggests, the main aim is not necessarily to develop policy-relevant recommendations but to contribute to theory, although of course such contributions are essential for an evidence-based understanding of how policy is likely to be implemented and what its consequences are. Although perhaps more inductive than framework analysis, grounded theory in practice involves a cyclical process of data collection, analysis, developing tentative theory, going back to do more data collection and analysis to test this out, and so on until the emerging theory is, to use Glaser and Strauss's term, 'saturated'. This means the point is reached at which the analysts are confident that they have a dense theory that is fully grounded in data that accounts for the complexity of the topic. It does not mean merely that 'no new themes emerged from the data'.

The first step in grounded theory is open coding, and intense, line-by-line analysis of the early data to answer the basic question 'what's going on?' There are a number of techniques for helping to do this, including:

- Looking for *in vivo* codes. These are the classifications that participants themselves use to 'divide up the world'. In Table 8.1, at line 129, the interviewee uses the phrase 'personal problems'. This is an *in vivo* code that suggests that there is a classification of the kinds of problems you might take to the doctor, and one category is 'personal problems'.
- Label all codes provisionally. As you begin to identify codes, these should be labelled. The process of thinking about what to call a category helps us identify what concept it refers to and moves away from a merely descriptive level.
- Asking a battery of questions about each line. For instance, if we just take lines 32 to 33 in the transcript in Table 8.1, we could ask: in what other situations might children have to help parents? Does 'has to go' mean that there is an expectation or an obligation? Does 'one of us' refer to the family, the children, or a broader community? What are the consequences of going/ not going? The aim is not necessarily to answer these questions but to generate a number of ideas for codes and evolving theories that will later be checked out in the data.

This intense coding is obviously not used for the whole data set but is a useful way of generating potential codes and ideas about the data. It is also a very useful process if you become 'stuck' with data analysis, as a way of generating some new directions to think about. As coding becomes more selective, it concentrates on the key codes that have been identified as core to the emerging theory.

A note on using computer software

A number of software packages now exist to help manage qualitative data. These packages do not *do* the analysis: the researcher still has to do the hard work of thinking about coding frameworks, attaching codes to data extracts and thinking about the relationships between those codes. However, on large projects, computer software can aid the tasks of managing the data and can help organize data and retrieve sections of them. Many packages have specific requirements for transcripts in terms of preferred layouts and conventions, so it is important to test a pilot section of your data before, for instance, having it all transcribed. One website with useful information and test versions of software is the CAQDAS (computer-aided qualitative data analysis software) Networking Project, at http://www.surrey.ac.uk/caqdas/.

Improving the quality of qualitative analysis

Whatever style of analysis you choose, it has to be done in such a way as to convince a reader that your interpretation is credible. This is perhaps particularly important if working in the field of health research, as many readers may be more familiar with more quantitative traditions and may have questions such as:

- How do I know these findings are not just the subjective interpretations of the researcher?
- How do I know the researchers haven't just picked out the examples that support their hypothesis?
- The sample is very small – how do I know these participants are representative of a larger population?

Analysis and writing has to be done with this kind of critic in mind: how can you convince them that your analysis was good enough to be credible? There are some criteria that describe good quality analysis and paying attention to these will help the credibility of your research. These are: comprehensiveness, thoroughness and transparency.

Comprehensiveness

Analysis should be systematic and comprehensive. If you are not coding all the data in detail, select the sample with clear criteria. When selecting quotes to illustrate points, make sure you note whether they are typical or unusual. Simple counts can help – instead of saying 'many people said x was the most important factor', say '10 of the 15 interviewed mentioned x as the most important factor'. Do not trawl the data to find examples that back up your theory but look at all the extracts under each thematic heading and make sure your interpretations account for all of them.

Thoroughness

As well as covering the whole data set, analysis should be thorough, fully accounting for variation with the data set and for the complexity of people's accounts. There are two key strategies for doing this: comparison and being critical.

Comparison

Analysis is driven by comparisons: between cases and within cases (do people say different things when talking about hypothetical cases and real experiences and do they make different explanations of events in their past history and their current practice?) and (if possible) between data sets (how do your findings differ from others on similar topics/similar populations?). Asking why things are the same or different is key to answering the basic question of 'what is going on here?'

One example from the bilingual young people's study was the comparison of stories in which young people said that interpreting was 'easy' and stories in which they talked about difficulties and problems. Examination of the two kinds of stories suggested some common features of 'easy' interpreting: it was more likely when children were younger (perhaps they were less aware of the problems) or when the consultation was for themselves rather than their parents, or when the consultation was for a routine problem when the outcome was agreed by all parties.

Being critical

Analysis should be approached in the spirit of testing emerging hypotheses, and constantly looking for disconfirming evidence. Credibility is enhanced if you have accounted for *deviant cases*: those examples that differ in significant ways from the rest of the data set. This could be, for instance, the one person who does not report a problem that all other participants mention, or for whom the consequences of an experience were different from those of other participants.

Transparency

If a reader can see exactly how you did your analysis, and what steps you took between data collection and interpretation, they can assess how far your conclusions are credible. Practical details and examples of coding decisions and how you came to agree on the main themes are more useful than general comments like 'we used grounded theory' or 'a framework analysis approach was used'.

Reliability

A basic prerequisite of credible research findings is that they were collected through rigorous research practice: accurate notes or interview transcripts were used, the topic guide was appropriate, and the interviewer was skilled in qualitative interviews. Good practice in analysis can also improve reliability.

Activity 8.4

Can you think of any ways of improving reliability in analysis?

Feedback

In some approaches, using more than one coder is a key way to improve reliability, especially early in the data analysis when codes are being defined. Some basic quantitative methods might also be useful, such as counting the frequency of certain behaviours, or themes in interviews. The development of computer software packages designed to aid qualitative data analysis has made this easier. Deliberately seeking negative cases, instead of being satisfied with the first 'good story' that emerges from the data, can aid the case that analysis methods used are reliable.

Generalizability

A common criticism of qualitative studies with small sample sizes is that they may not be generalizable. Methods such as participant observation require an intensive period of fieldwork and it is often not possible to include more than a small number of sites in the sample. Traditionally, ethnographies were based on a single site, studied in depth. Although this produces rich, detailed data about one setting, the findings may not be generalizable to others. Even in-depth interviews often cover a small number of respondents as the interviewing, transcribing and analysis are time consuming. Many studies reported in journals are based on 30 or fewer interviews and they may not be sampled as a representative group of the whole population.

Activity 8.5

In what ways do you think the results from participant observation or small qualitative interviews are generalizable? Think about the summary you read in Chapter 5 on the study of asthma patients. Could these findings be generalized more widely? Can you think of any ways of improving the generalizability of findings from qualitative studies?

Feedback

The aims of qualitative research are not to produce findings that are generalizable in a statistical sense but to produce *concepts* that are generalizable. In the example of the study of asthma patients, for instance, we do not know how far the proportions of patients in each group would represent a larger population, but we can find the broad typology generalizable. One test of theory in qualitative studies is how generalizable the concepts are: could you use them to help understand another setting? This typology might be useful in thinking about patients with other chronic problems.

The key to both the development of theory and generalizability is *comparison*, both within a set of data and between those data and other published work. It may be possible to find other settings reported in the literature that have similarities with the ones you have studied to provide comparative data.

The value of qualitative data is, then, not that it 'represents' in any statistical way the views of the whole population, or their behaviour, but that it can generate new concepts and theoretical insights. If can also *sensitize* practitioners or policy makers to potential issues of concern.

Summary

Qualitative analysis involves careful and theoretically informed coding to identify, in the data, indicators of underlying concepts that interest the researcher. Rigorous data collection and using more than one coder can improve reliability. Attention to theory (to how the concepts emerging from the data are connected and how they are examples of more general social situations) extends the generalizability of qualitative research.

References

Free C, Green J, Bhavnani V and Newman A (2003) Bilingual young people's experiences of interpreting in primary care: a qualitative study. *British Journal of General Practice* 53: 530–5.
Ritchie J and Spencer L (1994) Qualitative data analysis for applied policy research, in Bryman A and Burgess R-G (eds) *Analyzing Qualitative Data*. London: Routledge.
Strauss A (1987) *Qualitative Analysis for Social Scientists*. Cambridge: Cambridge University Press.

Further reading

Miles MB and Huberman AM (1994) *Qualitative Data Analysis: An Expanded Sourcebook* (2nd edn). Thousand Oaks, CA: Sage.

This is a very practical guide to the principles of analysis, and different ways of organizing, analysing and presenting qualitative data, which will appeal to those who like graphic aids to analysis such as grids and data matrices.

Seale C (1999) *The Quality of Qualitative Work*. London: Sage.

Clive Seale discusses various methodological positions on issues such as validity, reliability and generalizability and provides some practical approaches to maximizing the quality and credibility of qualitative analysis.

Strauss A and Corbin J (1990) *Basics of Qualitative Research: Grounded Theory Procedures and Techniques*. London: Sage.

This is an introduction to the processes of grounded theory for those relatively new to qualitative analysis, and many find it more readable than many texts on this approach.

9 | Practical: using qualitative methods

Judith Green

Overview

This chapter provides an opportunity to review the methods introduced in this section, and to gain some practical experience in one of them. For this chapter you are required to work through this text and to carry out some fieldwork. To complete the chapter, you will need the help of friends, family or work colleagues who may be your focus group research participants, or, if you decide to conduct an in-depth interview, the cooperation of four people who are not close friends, family or work colleagues.

The time taken to complete this practical will depend on how long the fieldwork takes. You may be able to combine fieldwork with your everyday working role. Thinking about the research question and writing up your notes should take about two hours.

Learning objectives

After working through this chapter, you will be better able to:

- **identify an appropriate strategy for collecting qualitative data**
- **use a strategy that you have selected to carry out qualitative research**

Choosing the research method

So far, you have studied a number of interview methods that can be used to generate qualitative data, including in-depth interviewing and focus groups. In this chapter, you will have an opportunity to carry out either interviews or focus groups. You will first choose a qualitative research question from some suggested topics and then decide which of these data collection strategies might appropriately generate useful data.

First, choose one of the following topics for your study:

- Patient satisfaction with one health provision with which you are familiar.
- Communication between different professional groups within a hospital or health centre: for instance, managers and doctors, or nurses and doctors.
- Infection control in a hospital or community setting.

Think of an aspect of the topic that is relevant to your own experience. From this, frame a qualitative research question and decide which data collection strategy will be most appropriate. Use the notes below as a guide to carrying out your data collection. Keep any notes you make, as you will need them again to inform your work in Chapter 13 when you design a survey instrument.

Guidance notes

In-depth interviews

Preparation

When you have decided on your research question, write a topic list to cover in the interview. Think of some 'open questions' that will generate more than a 'yes/no' answer, and some prompts (such as nods of the head or encouraging noises) you can use to get your respondents to expand on their answers. Also consider what kind of probes you might use to explore their answers.

Interviewing

Interview four people – if possible people who are not close friends, family or colleagues. Try to tape-record and transcribe a part of at least one interview, and make full notes of the others. When interviewing, remember to question in a non-judgemental and non-directive way. This can be very difficult if your professional background has trained you to ask directive questions, such as those used in a clinical interview. Remember that the aim is not to 'test' the respondents but to try to understand their way of seeing the world.

Reflection

Try coding part of the interviews. Are there common themes? Compare your own notes to the interview transcribed. What did you miss in your own notes? Can anything be added by considering the respondents' own words? Did the findings generate other research questions, or refine your own? Do you think you succeeded in understanding how respondents saw the world, and why?

Focus group

Preparation

Choose the participants you will invite. If you have willing work colleagues or friends, you might persuade them to give up an hour of their time in return for hospitality! A common experience is that of non-attendance, so invite more people than you need for the discussion. Make sure you have a room available where you won't be interrupted. You might want to plan some games or exercises to make participants feel comfortable with each other as well as generating data. Some to consider are:

- writing attitude statements on cards and asking the group to put them in order of strength of agreement

- asking participants to rank, for example, health services offered, in order of importance to them
- inviting them to share with a partner a 'critical incident', such as the best and worst aspect of their hospital stay, or working with other professions.

Consider whether you want all participants to contribute to the discussion, and how you could encourage this, or whether you want a more 'natural' discussion, and how this could be achieved. Think of the topics that you want the group to discuss, and some questions that will generate discussion.

Running the group

Introduce yourself and say why you are running the group. Explain how much time it will take and what the process will be. During the discussion, take notes of what is said and the reaction of other participants. Are there some topics that generate broad agreement? Are some opinions marginalized by the group? Are some topics sensitive?

Reflection

Did your group provide any data on how people interact? How would you run another group, if you were to repeat this exercise? What themes emerged as important for your participants? How useful were the data from any group exercises you ran?

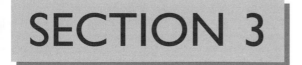

SECTION 3

Quantitative methods

Measurement in the social sciences

John Browne and Judith Green

Overview

This chapter introduces issues in quantitative research through a discussion of some of the principles of measurement. Good measurement techniques are essential for good quantitative research; however well designed a quantitative study is, it will not answer the research question if we have not designed appropriate, precise and reliable instruments. This is an area of methodology most associated with the discipline of psychology, in which much of the good work on measurement in the social sciences has been generated.

Learning objectives

After working through this chapter you will be better able to:

- **distinguish between nominal, ordinal, ratio and interval measurement scales**
- **appreciate the role of theory in measurement**
- **identify different kinds of validity and reliability in quantitative research**

Key terms

Measurement scale The level of measurement used (nominal, ordinal, ratio, interval).

Reliability The extent to which an instrument produces consistent results.

Validity The extent to which an indicator measures what it intends to measure.

Introduction

Qualitative methods are particularly well suited to research that seeks to understand people's behaviour or the meanings they attribute to the social world. However, public health professionals can also gain understanding of their research topic from quantitative research (research that involves numerical measurement). Often qualitative and quantitative research will be used in a complementary fashion to increase understanding (see Chapter 16).

In the examples examined in the chapters in the previous section on qualitative research, it might be important to follow up qualitative research with studies that *measure* some of the variables identified as important. For instance, in the example of focus groups used to investigate the views of south Asians with diabetes (Chapter 7) you might need to know how many south Asians need information written in languages other than English and which languages are needed. You might need to know how many south Asians have been diagnosed as diabetic in different areas of Britain, in order to plan services, or what level of underdiagnosis is likely, so that you can assess unmet need.

A range of quantitative methods are used in social sciences. The most common are based on either the analysis of existing statistics, on specially commissioned surveys of samples of the population or on investigations using controlled conditions. This section concentrates on these kinds of methods, although of course there are many other quantitative approaches used in the social sciences, including content analysis of texts and documents (in which the number of times particular themes or issues occurring in the text is counted) and quantitative approaches to observational work, involving counting the occurrence of particular behaviours.

Policy makers, managers and front-line professionals increasingly rely on quantitative data about the population they serve, their health problems and how the health care system itself functions. This chapter will help you understand the theory of measurement and the importance of developing valid and reliable quantitative indicators.

Statistics

In the early nineteenth century in northern Europe, governments began to collect increasing numbers of 'facts' about their populations. Since then, across most of the world, state governments and their departments have gathered ever more sophisticated measurements of their citizens. As individuals, we are now the objects of considerable surveillance, with details about our homes, health, use of health services, consumer preferences, and views collected not only by government agencies and public bodies, but also commercial organizations. The health service manager, like managers in any other public or private organization, relies on an increasing range of quantified data to monitor and plan their work. This includes the 'routine statistics' collated by other people, as well as the information that they themselves produce.

Activity 10.1

What sources of quantified data does your workplace use or collect?

↻ **Feedback**

> If you are working in a hospital, managers may routinely collect data about the number of patients resident, their demographic characteristics (for example, date of birth, post-code, gender, ethnicity), their length of stay, the number of staff at different grades, the treatment activities undertaken (such as number of hip replacements performed per year) and the costs of care. Hospital professionals may also routinely collect clinical and other data about their patients, which may be collated to contribute to national data sets. This clinical data are likely to include measures of pre-treatment morbidity (such as stage of cancer), comorbidity (other diseases and disorders the patient may have) and outcomes (such as symptom alleviation after treatment, mortality). In addition, sources of information collected by others, such as local population estimates, may be used by hospitals to anticipate local needs.

Quantitative research methods

In almost every area of life we contribute to quantitative data collection or use data collected by others. The quantitative social sciences have their roots in this growth of 'official statistics' and have developed a number of techniques for quantifying, or 'measuring', aspects of social life. Quantitative techniques involve the use of standardized and scheduled questionnaires, rather than the more open methods discussed in Chapters 5 to 9. Methods of analysis rely on manipulation of numerical data, rather than textual analysis. Survey research concentrates on generalities and on 'normality' (in a statistical sense) and departures from it, rather than the in-depth investigation of a particular case or setting that sometimes characterizes qualitative research. However, the contrast between quantitative and qualitative methods should not be exaggerated (these are tendencies, rather than absolute descriptions), and they are often best used in combination.

Chapter 11 describes what is perhaps the most widely used data collection tool in the social sciences, the questionnaire. Chapter 12 introduces what is perhaps the most widely used quantitative research design in the social sciences, the survey. Before studying how to design questionnaires and use them in surveys, it is important to understand something about what is meant by 'measurement' and how you can ensure that instruments used in research are as reliable and valid as possible.

Much of the work in the theory of measurement and validity in the social sciences has come from the discipline of *psychometric testing*, in which psychologists have developed techniques for assessing outcomes such as 'quality of life' and for testing instruments to demonstrate that they are reliable and valid. Although you may never have to design a health outcome instrument, the principles of this discipline are useful for framing a more general discussion of measurement in quantitative research.

Measurement

In previous chapters, it was suggested that qualitative methods could be used to explore how people *classify* the world: how, for instance, they understand concepts such as health. An in-depth understanding of what is meant by such abstract terms as 'quality of life' or 'social class' is essential, as you have seen, to clarify what indicators are needed to investigate them. In quantitative research, the aim is to 'measure' these indicators in order to answer questions such as:

'How much x is there in the population?'
'Is there more x than y?'
'To what extent is x larger than y?'

These questions imply different levels of measurement. Measurement scales are conventionally divided into four kinds, depending on what kind of categories are used to classify the variable being measured and what assumptions can be made about the relationships between these categories. These assumptions have implications for the kinds of statistical analysis that can be done on the resulting data. The four levels of measurement are:

- **Nominal**. This is the most basic level of measurement, which involves merely classifying and labelling (*naming*) two or more categories (such as eye colour, occupation or diagnosis), without making any assumptions about their relative value. A hospital survey that counted how many inpatients were resident in the surgical, medical, and maternity wards would be 'measuring' patients on the nominal scale of 'specialty'. If data are at the nominal level, they can be used to compare distribution across the categories (for instance, to compare the number of surgical and medical patients in any one week) and statistical tests can be applied to see if the distribution is 'normal', or one that would be expected.
- **Ordinal**. An ordinal scale not only labels the categories of interest, but also ranks them in an *order*. To help work out staffing arrangements, a nurse managing a ward might categorize his or her patients in three groups of their dependency, from 'fully independent', 'needs some help in self care' to 'needs help for all self-care tasks'. Although this scale of 'dependency' does not measure how much more dependent a patient in one group is than another, it does rank them in order.
- **Interval**. An interval scale has more information in that it not only ranks the categories of interest but ranks them in such a way that there is a known difference between them, although the starting point of the scale (the 0 on a numerical scale) is arbitrary. Temperature measured in Celsius is a well-known example of an interval scale. Although the difference between 5 °C and 10 °C may be the same as that between 25 °C and 30 °C, because the *interval* between the two measures is the same (5°), the beginning of the scale is arbitrary (and different from that used if we were measuring in Fahrenheit). The absence of a 'real' starting point means that we can only answer questions such as 'how much hotter is x than y?' It would be a nonsense to say 'patient x was twice as hot as patient y'.
- **Ratio**. The strongest measurement scale has an absolute starting-point (zero), so not only can the distances between points on the scale be compared but they can be compared proportionally, or by *ratios*. Thus, 'cost' is usually measured on a ratio scale, by attributing a price. Prices can then not only be compared in

absolute terms but also in terms of proportion. If, for instance, the average cost of a day surgery procedure is £500, whereas that for inpatient care is £2000, it is possible to say that inpatient care costs four times as much as day care. In a ratio scale, the unit of measurement (whether it is pounds, dollars or any other currency) does not affect the ratio between two measurements. In this example, inpatient care would still cost four times more if it were measured in US dollars. If the characteristic of interest can be measured on a ratio scale, this enables the researcher to use more powerful statistics to investigate the distribution of variables within the population and relationships between them. However, in the social sciences the concepts we are interested in are often only measurable at a lower level.

✎ **Activity 10.2**

Four items from a questionnaire used to survey hospital inpatients are listed. Alongside each one, note what level of measurement is being used to rate the responses.

1) Are you male or female? (circle one)
2) How many days did you stay in the hospital? _____ days
3) On a scale of 1 (no pain at all) to 10 (extreme pain), how would you rate your pain level on the day you were discharged? (circle one number)

   1   2   3   4   5   6   7   8   9   10

4) How satisfied were you with cleanliness of your ward? (circle one answer)

   Very satisfied   Satisfied   Neutral   Dissatisfied   Very dissatisfied

---

↻ **Feedback**

1) Gender is measured on a *nominal* scale. By convention, there are usually just two categories called 'male' and 'female'.

2) Length of stay is measured on a *ratio* scale, with number of days. If patients had instead been given the following choices:

- less than 2 days
- between 2 and 5 days
- more than 5 days

the scale would have been *ordinal*.

3) This scale is a really an *ordinal* scale, as there is no way of knowing whether the points are equidistant. However, response scales like this are sometimes treated as *interval* data for statistical analysis (the distance between the points is assumed to be the same). The extent to which this assumption is tolerated depends among other things on the number of points on the scale: a 10-point scale is often treated as though it were interval, but it would be very rare to treat a three-point scale in this fashion.

4) This is an *ordinal* scale, where the response categories are merely ranked in order.

Role of theory in social science measurements

In biomedical sciences measurement poses fewer problems than perhaps it does for social scientists. There are a number of reasons for this:

- There is greater clarity over the concepts to be measured (for example, height, weight, cholesterol levels).
- There are agreed indicators for measuring many of these concepts (for example, 'amount of mercury pushed up a tube' for blood pressure).
- There are reliable and valid measurement instruments (such as the thermometer for temperature)
- There are also agreed units of measurement, which are usually at least at the interval level.

This does not imply that there are no problems in the biomedical sciences, however. For many of the concepts of interest (such as 'fitness for surgery', 'extent of comorbidity') there are problems with the indicators that have been developed in some or all of the areas mentioned above.

In the social sciences, because the concepts used are more abstract, it may be much more difficult to develop appropriate indicators, and they are more likely to be at the nominal or ordinal level. Compare, for instance, the debate about how to measure 'intelligence' with the agreement about how to measure temperature. The problem is not just that there is no equivalent to the thermometer to use but that there is considerable disagreement about what intelligence *is*, and what might be appropriate indicators of it:

- scores on an IQ test which measures non-verbal reasoning
- skills in 'real-life' problem solving or
- educational qualifications gained.

For this reason, indicators for many concepts used in health research reflect an underlying theory of what the concept is and how it is related to other concepts. Theory has an important bearing on how indicators are chosen, whether the researcher is designing a psychometric outcome measure or a questionnaire for a more general survey. In her survey of the health of the population of Britain, Mildred Blaxter (1990) had to consider 'what is health?' in order to develop ways of operationalizing it for measurement.

Activity 10.3

Read the following extract by Mildred Blaxter (1990) and note down answers to the following questions:

1) Why did Blaxter ask respondents to her survey to define the concept of health?
2) Why could 'health' not be defined in terms of 'deviations of measurable biological variables from the norm'?
3) How does Blaxter contrast the social science survey methodology she uses to 'classic epidemiology'?

📖 Health and Lifestyles (introduction)

In 1984/5 a large national survey of the population of England, Wales and Scotland, the Health and Lifestyle Survey, was carried out. In it, people were asked in great detail about their health and lifestyles, certain aspects of their fitness were measured, and they were invited to express their opinion and attitudes towards health and health related behaviour . . .

First, health must be defined. There are no simple or obvious ways in which this can be done . . . Disease or physiological status can be identified or measured . . . but this is not the whole of health: health and illness are social as well as biological facts . . .

In the biomedical model on which much of modern medicine is based, disease is defined as deviations of measurable biological variables from the norm, or the presence of defined and categorized forms of pathology . . .

The respondents to this survey demonstrated clearly that 'health', more widely defined, was for them essentially a relative state, influences notably by the normal aging process. Health could be identified as simply the absence of disease, but for most people it was more than that, They tended to agree, it would seem, with the World Health Organization's definition of health as 'a state of complete physical, social and mental well being and not merely the absence of disease or infirmity' . . .

Trying to operationalize such a wide concept of health has the danger of subsuming all human life and happiness under this label: nevertheless it does draw attention to the fact that positive aspects of healthiness ought to be considered . . .

The definition of health used in this study, therefore, is essentially multi-dimensional and relative. It includes both objective and subjective components, and attempts to consider the positive as well as negative range . . .

The . . . era of classical epidemiology focused, with great success, upon diseases – whether caused by micro-organisms, or viruses, nutrient deficiencies, toxins or other causative agents – where the model of a specific agent, giving rise to a specific disease, seemed appropriate.

The traditional approaches of epidemiology become more complex, however, in the modern Western world, where many of the health problems are degenerative and chronic. There is now recognition that most diseases have multiple and interactive causes . . . More complex – if at the same time less precise and demonstrable – levels of explanation may be required. (1990: 1–4)

↻ Feedback

1) Blaxter argues that there is no accepted definition of health, and that it is defined as a *social* as well as a biological fact, so it is necessary to take 'lay' definitions into account.

2) Although 'absence of disease', which such deviations imply, was one important element of health, most people had a broader definition which included feelings of positive wellbeing.

3) This survey does not address the causes or prevalence of specific diseases, and could not do so. Instead, by using a multi-dimensional definition of health, which included measures of fitness, questions about lifestyle behaviours, questions about health-related attitudes and questions about social circumstances, the survey can be used to explore the relationships between behaviour, attitudes, circumstances and health.

Validity

The problem of operationalizing variables was introduced in Chapter 3, and it was noted that choice of indicator often involved a compromise, as concepts in social science are seldom easily measured. *Validity* refers to how well the indicator or, more usually, indicators, that have been chosen do actually measure the underlying concept. The validity of the measure depends on the 'fit' between the concept and the indicators chosen. A single indicator will rarely be adequate. Concepts such as 'health' or 'intelligence' are multi faceted, so more faith can be placed in a measurement strategy that uses a variety of indicators, each one operationalizing a different aspect of the concept, than in one that relies on only a single indicator of a concept. Thus, in Blaxter's *Health and Lifestyles* survey, the researchers identified four dimensions of health, and a set of indicators to measure each dimension. They are shown in Table 10.1.

Table 10.1 Four dimensions of health

Dimension of concept	Indicators
Fitness	Physiological measurements
Absence of disease/impairment	Reported medically defined conditions
Experienced freedom from illness	Reports of symptoms suffered
Psychosocial wellbeing	Reports of psychosocial symptoms

Source: Blaxter (1990)

The issue of validity is as important in quantitative work as in qualitative work and it refers to the same general issues: how can the reader have faith in the 'truth' of the researcher's account? In quantitative research, though, there are more formal methods that can help demonstrate validity. Unfortunately, there is never one piece of evidence which can demonstrate conclusively that a measure is valid. Validity cannot be 'proved' but there are ways of improving the credibility of quantitative indicators. These are essential tools not only for researchers who need to reassure themselves that they are using an appropriate instrument but also for readers and users of research, who need to consider the validity of indicators chosen.

Types of validity

In your reading, you may encounter different terminology to describe validity across the social science disciplines. However, the underlying principles are the same. Streiner and Norman (2003) describe it thus:

> Validation is a process of hypothesis testing: 'Someone who scores high on this measure will also do well in situation A, perform poorly on test B and will differ from those who score low on the scale on traits C and D'.

What is more important is that you understand the following ideas, rather than remembering the various names for different kinds of validity used by those working in psychometric testing and theory. Taken together, these various sources can strengthen the credibility of the measure used.

Face validity

This is the most straightforward measure of validity, and relies on whether the indicator 'looks like' it is a measure of the variable of interest. Clearly this can never be an adequate measure on its own as our subjective judgements about measures are likely to be partial and biased. However, using a panel of colleagues, perhaps, to look over an instrument would provide useful information about its 'face validity'.

Content validity

This refers to the representativeness of the range of indicators chosen to measure a concept. Content validity is high when a scale (a set of items) includes components that cover all the elements of the concept it is intended to measure. For example, we would expect a symptom checklist for patients undergoing cancer chemo-therapy to include a wide range of symptoms that arise in this situation, and not just focus on one or two symptoms.

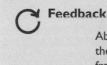

Activity 10.4

Why would self-reports of disease diagnosis be inadequate for Blaxter's *Health and Lifestyles* survey, in terms of content validity?

Feedback

Absence of disease would not have been a complete measure of 'health', because the theoretical concept of health used in this survey covered other dimensions (fitness, freedom from symptoms, psychosocial wellbeing) as well as 'absence of disease'.

Criterion validity

This refers to the extent to which the indicator chosen correlates with some other (known to be valid) indicator of the concept. Thus, to know if the questionnaire item 'How many units of alcohol have you drunk today?' was a valid measure of daily alcohol intake, it might be possible to correlate answers with measurements of blood alcohol levels as a 'gold standard' indicator of alcohol intake. Here, 'blood alcohol level' is the *criterion* by which the questionnaire item is being measured. It is important to understand, however, that there are rarely, if ever, true 'gold standard' indicators for the things we are trying to measure; there are just indicators where there is more-or-less agreement (based on more-or-less valid-ity testing) on the extent to which they measure what they are supposed to measure.

Construct validity

In the social sciences there is often poor agreement over what constitutes a 'gold standard' indicator, and often there will be agreement that there is nothing approaching a gold standard. Thus it can be difficult to demonstrate criterion validity. In addition (as in the previous example on alcohol intake) it may simply not be possible (for ethical or other reasons) to test it in this way.

An alternative approach is to use construct validation. Here we attempt to measure whether the indicator performs in the way that the underlying theory says it should. To do this we must first generate hypotheses about our concept. Let us use the example of a questionnaire (the indicator) designed to measure the quality of life of people with cancer (the concept). The following are some of the types of hypotheses we might generate about how the questionnaire should perform: known groups differences; convergence with related indicator; lack of convergence with unrelated indicators.

- *Known groups*. We might expect patients with more advanced cancer, or those on treatments with serious side effects to have lower quality of life scores on the questionnaire than patients with early cancer stages and no treatment side effects.
- *Convergence*. We might expect scores on our questionnaire to correlate positively with related indicators, such as measures of physical or mental health.
- *Lack of convergence (also known as discriminant validity)*. Unless part of our theory, we would not expect women, for example, to have lower scores than men. We would also hope that our questionnaire does not correlate too highly with personality measures, such as the tendency to give socially desirable responses.

One of the main problems with construct validations is the uncertainty over the status of your theoretical assumptions. If, for example, we find that women score lower on our quality of life questionnaire, is this a problem with our questionnaire or our theory?

Reliability

When we design a measurement instrument we want to be able to detect the 'true' state of the concept of interest, and we want to be able to detect differences in that concept. These may be differences between people or things (for example, differences in body weight of different patient groups) or differences over time (such as differences in average temperature from year to year).

There are two main reasons why our concepts may differ. If we take the example of weighing scales as an indicator of the concept 'weight over time', the data produced by the scales may differ from day to day because (a) our weight changes from day to day and (b) the weighing scales have a certain amount of random variation, which influences the weight reading over and above any changes in our daily weight. This random variation is an undesirable interference, or 'noise' which reduces our confidence in the accuracy of our data.

The term 'reliability' is often used interchangeably with consistency, stability and repeatability but these are often confusing to those unfamiliar with the true concept of reliability. The term 'stability' for example seems to suggest that we do not want the data from our measurement instrument to change over time. This is obviously not true: scales would be useless if they told you that you weighed the same every day, even while you are putting on weight!

Reliability may therefore be best thought of as the proportion of differences in measurements due to *true* differences in the concept being measured, having accounted for random variations (errors) in the measurement instrument. The higher the proportion of change in our measurement data that is due to 'true' difference, the more reliable our measurement instrument.

In quantitative research, instruments such as survey questionnaires can be statistically *tested* for reliability, to see that they are unaffected by the rater (such as the interviewer) used, or the setting.

There are two major aspects to testing the reliability of instruments:

- *Test-retest reliability* – this is the extent to which the instrument is stable over time, given that nothing has changed in the concept of interest over that time period. It can be tested by asking respondents to complete the same form at two different times when no change is expected.
- *Inter-rater/observer reliability* – if the questionnaire or schedule relies on an interviewer or other rater to complete, it can be tested to see that different raters record the same responses in the same way (that the data produced are not influenced by the rater producing them).

Activity 10.5

Read the following summary of two studies (Baker 1990 and Baker and Whitfield 1992) used to develop questionnaire instruments for assessing patient satisfaction with general practitioners in the UK, and note how they tried to ensure the validity and reliability of their measures.

Developing a patient satisfaction questionnaire

Although the importance of assessing patient satisfaction with care is widely recognized, there are no well-validated instruments that have been tested for use with patients in the UK. Richard Baker and his colleagues developed two instruments to investigate how satisfied patients were with the consultations they had with their doctor (the Consultation Satisfaction Questionnaire, or CSQ) and how satisfied they were with the surgery in general (the Surgery Satisfaction Questionnaire, or SSQ). They began by reviewing other work on patient satisfaction to identify the dimensions that might contribute to the concept 'satisfaction' and talking to professionals and patients about their experiences of care. A preliminary list of statements to cover these dimensions was drawn up, some worded positively (for example, 'This doctor examined me very thoroughly') and some negatively (for example, 'The time I was able to spend with the doctor was a bit too short'). Colleagues were asked to comment on the meaning of the items included and the questionnaires were piloted on patients to identify any ambiguous or leading questions and to ask if they wanted to make any other comments on satisfaction with their doctor.

Revised lists of statements were then tested with patients. Results from these surveys were analysed statistically in order to look for correlations between the different items, in order to identify 'factors', or dimensions of patient satisfaction (groups of items that were generally answered in similar ways). This suggested three main factors, which the researchers called professional care, depth of relationship and perceived time.

On testing the Consultation Satisfaction Questionnaire, they found that it discriminated between different doctors in that there were statistically significant differences in the scores each received on the three dimensions of the CSQ. A further study was carried out, in which SSQ and the CSQ were found to discriminate in the predicted direction between a group of patients who had changed GP (and so could be assumed to be dissatisfied with the care they received) and those who had not. Discuss all the kinds of validity that the researchers were interested in here. What kind of validity were they unable to establish?

Feedback

These are some of the kinds of validity that you may have discussed:

- Reviewing other work and asking patients about satisfaction with care maximizes *content validity*, in that the researchers could be fairly confident that there were items covering the major dimensions of their concept.
- Asking colleagues to judge whether the items look reasonable is a measure of *face validity*.
- They were not able to look at *criterion validity*, because there were no 'gold standard' measures currently in use in the UK.
- Instead, *construct validity* was tested to see if the measure adequately measured lower satisfaction in a group of patients who had chosen to change doctors and whether it distinguished between different doctors.

In the quantitative social sciences, considerations of validity often presuppose that there is one underlying 'truth' about, for instance, health status or satisfaction. Using blood alcohol measures as a test of criterion validity of a questionnaire measure of alcohol intake presupposes, for instance, that blood alcohol readings are a 'true' measure of alcohol intake.

Activity 10.6

Think back to the discussion of different approaches to science in Chapter 2, when different perspectives on social science methodology were discussed. How would you characterize the approach to validity described in the above paragraph?

Feedback

It is a positivist approach, because there is an implicit assumption that there is one 'reality' of alcohol intake, and that the proper role of social science methods is to refine our ways of measuring it.

Summary

In quantitative social science research, the aim is to 'measure' concepts such as social and behavioural characteristics, respondents' attitudes and their beliefs. Measurement poses problems because the concepts social scientists work with are complex, multidimensional and can be difficult to operationalize. Indicators have to be theoretically informed. The social science discipline of psychometric theory and testing has made a major contribution to the theory of measurement and the testing of validity. When using findings from quantitative work, it is necessary to ask whether the researchers have demonstrated the reliability and validity of the indicators they have chosen. In the next chapter, the principles of questionnaire design are outlined.

References

Baker R (1990) Development of a questionnaire to assess patients' satisfaction with consultations in general practice. *British Journal of General Practice* 40: 487–90.

Baker R and Whitfield M (1992) Measuring patient satisfaction: a test of construct validity. *Quality in Health Care* 1: 104–9.

Blaxter M (1990) *Health and Lifestyles*. London: Tavistock.

Streiner DL and Norman GR (2003) *Health Measurement Scales: A Practical Guide to Their Development and Use* (3rd edn). Oxford: Oxford University Press.

Further reading

Bowling A (1997) *Measuring Health: A Review of Quality of Life Measurement Scales* (2nd edn). Milton Keynes: Open University Press.

McClure RJ, Peel N, Kassulke D, Neale R (2002) Appropriate indicators for injury control? *Public Health* 116: 252–6.

Finding appropriate indicators for health research is challenging. Bowling (1997) is a general review of health measurements issues; McClure *et al.* (2002) deals with the problem for one particular area, that of injury control.

Questionnaire design

John Browne

Overview

There are many pitfalls for the novice questionnaire designer. Designing good, reliable and valid questionnaires is a skilled task and is more difficult than it might look. As a public health practitioner or health services manager, you may need to design simple questionnaires yourself, and you will need some skills in assessing those designed by other researchers. This chapter introduces the principles of questionnaire design.

Learning objectives

After working through this chapter, you will be better able to:

- **identify some common problems when designing a questionnaire**
- **understand the principles of good questionnaire design**

Key terms

Closed question Question which gives the respondent a predetermined choice of responses.

Open question Question that allows the respondent to give any answer.

Should you carry out a questionnaire survey?

A questionnaire is a structured schedule used to elicit predominantly quantitative data. It can be completed by the respondent (a self-completed questionnaire), or can be used verbally, by an interviewer reading out the questions to the respondent. Questionnaires have a wide range of uses in health and health services research, including:

- population surveys, such as the *Health and Lifestyles* survey described in Activity 10.3
- management evaluations of user satisfaction with services
- outcomes research, in which psychometric questionnaires are developed to provide patient-based evaluations of such constructs as quality of life.

Like any other method of data collection, questionnaires have a number of advantages and disadvantages.

Advantages

Written or Internet-based questionnaires are very cost-effective when compared to face-to-face interviews. Questionnaires are also very easy to analyse provided they address clearly formulated research questions. Data entry and tabulation can be done with computer software packages, which can also reduce the time and money required. Questionnaires are familiar and non-threatening to most people as nearly everyone has had some experience completing them. Questionnaires also have the potential to reduce researcher bias because each question is presented uniformly (this does not guarantee, however, that questions will be interpreted in a uniform fashion by respondents). Finally, postal, or Internet questionnaires are generally not as time consuming or intrusive as interviews or focus groups: respondents can complete them when they please, providing they meet the response deadline.

Disadvantages

One major disadvantage of postal questionnaires is the lack of control over responses. Response rates as low as 10% can occur with poorly designed surveys, which reduces our ability to trust the representativeness of the results. It is even possible that the person completing an anonymous questionnaire may not be the person to whom it was sent. Even if people do send their questionnaires back, it is possible that many questions may have been missed or answered in an incorrect fashion (for example, by ticking more than one box when only one response is allowed). This may be due to poor design but it is also common that some respondents have reading and comprehension difficulties. Another disadvantage of questionnaires is the inflexible nature of such a structured instrument. For example, a questionnaire might reveal that respondents are dissatisfied with their job, but the exact source of that dissatisfaction may be much harder to discover. In an interview we can directly ask 'what is it that you dislike about your job', but in a questionnaire we may have to provide a long list of options, which may take a long time to work through and still not capture the exact flavour of the problem. By allowing free space for comments one can address this problem, but free text responses are difficult to tabulate, and undermine one of the main advantages of a questionnaire (ease of interpretation).

Project design

Most problems with questionnaires can be traced to uncertainty over the goals of the project. You should begin by writing out what you want to discover, and then generating questions that address these issues. One of the best ways to further clarify your study goals is to decide how you intend to analyse each piece of information in your questionnaire. Longer questionnaires tend to have lower response rates: ask only questions that directly address the study goals and avoid the temptation to ask questions because it would be 'interesting to know'. As with any piece of research you should take time to operationalize the variables under study carefully, as we discussed in Chapter 3.

Generating questions

The first task when generating questions is to choose the variables you want to measure. There are many ways to do this. You may take a purely theoretical approach. Imagine that you are a manager at a hospital where staff absenteeism is considered too high and you have decided to carry out a questionnaire survey of staff to find out why. You might ask about job satisfaction, worker stress or child-care needs in your survey because your theory predicts these are important determinants of absenteeism. It is unlikely however that you will anticipate all important issues relevant to your research question on the basis of theory alone. A second useful way to identify important variables to be included is focus group discussions and/or interviews with key informants. You might ask hospital staff (in a focus group or in one-on-one interviews), for example, why they think people are leaving. A third way of identifying important variables might be a literature review. It is likely that research in other health care settings has already been carried out, and if you are lucky there may be other questionnaires on staff turnover that you can use rather than having to design one yourself. However, these will need to be checked carefully to make sure they are appropriate in your setting. At a minimum, even if the instrument is in the language you need, this will include checking that vocabulary is appropriate to the context. For instance, terms such as 'Nurse Manager' or 'Department' are likely to have different meanings in different hospitals. Ideally, an instrument should be validated for any new population with which it will be used.

Once you have chosen the variables to be addressed you must define these variables in a manner that can be used in a questionnaire. This has implications for both the 'question' and 'response' for each item in our questionnaire. To continue our example, if we want to ask our hospital staff directly about their recent absenteeism we must first define absenteeism so that the 'question' is clear. Do we mean absent from work for any reason; absent for all non-health reason or absent only for health reasons? What is the time period we are referring to (for example, last month, 3 months, 12 months and so on)? The choice of this period depends on both our own research question, and what we think is feasible (for instance, if we ask about the last 12 months this might confuse new employees hired within that period or it might be difficult to accurately recall absenteeism over 12 months).

We must then decide how to represent levels of absenteeism in the 'response' part of our question. Should we use an open-ended response format (such as 'How many days have you missed from work for any reason (not including annual leave) in the last 3 months? Please specify number _____ '). Or should we use a closed format (such as 'How many days have you missed from work for any reason (not including annual leave) in the last 3 months? Please circle one of the following: 0, 1, 2, 3, 4, 5, 6, more than 6'). If we choose a closed format, should we use numbers as in the previous example, or use non-numerical categories? The latter might be more suited to questions where exact numbers are not appropriate for the variables in question (for example, 'How would you describe your stress levels at work in the last year: severe, moderate, mild, none?'). In summary, questions and response choices need to be constructed so that respondents can be successful in giving answers that meet the analytic needs of the inquiry.

What makes a good question?

When we ask a question in a questionnaire, we hope that our respondents will answer accurately and honestly. There are a number of psychological processes that can inhibit accuracy and honesty.

Excess mental demands

Streiner and Norman (2003) describe the steps that respondents go through when answering a questionnaire. At each of these steps, accuracy can be impaired because the questionnaire places too much demand on important mental processes. It is imperative, therefore, that we try to minimize the mental demands on our respondents:

- *Misunderstanding the question.* Simple misunderstanding of the intention behind a question is very common. In the next section we describe many ways of minimizing misunderstandings, but some mismatch between questionnaire designer and respondent is always likely to exist.
- *Inability to recall.* If we ask people 'how satisfied have you been with work over the last year?' we are asking them to recall many moods and events over a long period, an extremely difficult task.
- *Guessing.* The answers to many of our questions cannot be recalled with perfect accuracy so our respondents must use a variety of strategies to 'guess' what they consider to be the 'right' answer. Streiner and Norman discuss a number of processes that can lead to errors in these guesses.
- *Mapping the answer onto the response alternative.* Response formats are unlikely to correspond exactly to our respondents' individual mental representations, and the 'true' answer can often become lost in translation. For example, we might provide the response choices 'excellent', 'very good', 'good', 'fair' and 'poor' to a question on subjective health, but our respondents might not consider the discrimination between 'excellent' and 'very good' to be valid for their own health, or they might want the option of describing their health as 'very poor'.

Biased responses

The second main problem for questionnaire designers arises from a variety of biases that occur when answering questions:

- *Satisficing.* This occurs when respondents give what they consider a 'satisfactory' rather than optimal answer. A common example of this is the tendency to select the first response alternative that seems reasonable, rather than considering all options and then choosing.
- *Social desirability and faking good.* Respondents are likely to want to present the best version of themselves to the world in a questionnaire. This can lead to extreme bias when we ask about, for example, socially undesirable behaviours (for example, illegal drug use).
- *Deviation and faking bad.* There are some situations where the respondent may perceive that it is advantageous to appear in as bad a light as possible. For instance, in a survey of adolescents, young men might exaggerate their experiences of alcohol use or smoking, if these are acceptable among their peer groups.

- *Acquiescence*. There is some evidence to suggest that respondents are more likely to agree than disagree with statements in a questionnaire. This is particularly problematic when we are asking about opinions or attitudes.
- *End-avoidance and positive skew*. These problems all arise when respondents are asked to provide an answer on some form of continuous scale. End avoidance occurs because respondents often do not like to choose extreme answers. Positive skew occurs because respondents tend to favour more positive responses, leading to response distributions that do not centre on the middle option.

Individual question tips

Given what we have learned about the psychological processes involved in answering questions, let us now consider some of the qualities of a good question. These include:

- Neutral wording. Value-laden questions produce biased responses.
- It avoids asking two or more questions at the same time.
- It accommodates all possible answers.
- It has mutually exclusive response choices, so that a single answer cannot fall into more than one category.
- There are unambiguous differences between the response choices.
- It produces variability of responses. When a question produces no variability in responses, we learn little from the question and cannot perform any statistical analyses on the item.
- It does not make unwarranted assumptions.
- It does not ask questions where the respondent has to guess (satisfice) the correct answer.
- It does not imply a desired answer. The wording of a question is extremely important. We are striving for objectivity in our surveys and, therefore, must be careful not to lead the respondent into giving the answer we would like to receive. Leading questions are usually easily spotted because they use negative phraseology. The exception to this is perhaps where we might expect social desirability to bias responses, and a leading question (implying, for instance, that most respondents did have this experience) may be more likely to generate an honest answer.

Activity 11.1

Imagine that we have constructed our questionnaire on hospital staff absenteeism. Using the individual question tips above, try to identify the errors present in each of the following questions that we have generated.

1   How would you describe your relationship with your line manager?
    Excellent/ Very good/ Good/ Average/ Fair/ Poor/ Very poor
2   Which type of co-worker do you find it most difficult to work with?
    Nursing staff/ Medical staff/ Management/ Other (please specify)
3   Do you ever miss work for child care or health reasons?
    Yes/No

4   Do you feel that you have received enough training in communicating with the relatives of recently deceased patients?
    Yes/No
5   Have you ever considered moving to a new job?
    Yes/No
6   How many days have you missed from work (for any reason, other than annual leave) in the last 12 months?
    1–5 days/ 6–10 days/ 11–15 days/ 16–20 days
7   Do you often miss work for no good reason?
    Yes/No
8   Isn't it true that flexible working hours are likely to improve staff morale?
    Yes/No
9   How many times have you felt very tired at work in the last month?
    0/ 1/ 2/ 3/ 4/ 5/ 6/ 7/ 8/ 9/ 10/ more than 10

↻ Feedback

Has ambiguous differences between the response choice (what is the difference between 'average' and 'fair'?)

May have response choices that are not mutually exclusive, because in a hospital many of the management may also be nurses or medical professionals.

Would be better as two questions. We would probably like to be able to separate out poor health and lack of child care as sources of absenteeism.

May make unwarranted assumptions – perhaps the respondent never has to deal with the relatives of recently deceased patients. One might be tempted to introduce a 'branching' question ('Do you deal with the relatives of recently deceased patients? Yes/No. If yes, please proceed . . .' and so forth). However, as a rule, branching in written questionnaires should be avoided because it sometimes confuses respondents. A better alternative might be to simply have the following response alternatives: 'Yes/No/ I do not deal with the relatives of recently deceased patients'.

Is unlikely to produce a variability of responses. It would be a rare employee that has not thought of moving to a new job.

Has broad enough categories that we can feel confident the respondent does not have to guess the answer (although they might find it difficult to be 100% confident about answers around the boundaries of the categories). The main problem is the lack of a zero option, or an option for those who have missed more than 20 days work.

Is value laden. The phrase 'no good reason' has strong negative connotations and is likely to encourage respondents to 'fake good'.

Is leading. The question 'Isn't it true . . .?' seems to encourage the respondent to agree with some conventional wisdom.

Imposes high demands on the respondent's memory and is likely to lead to guessing.

Overall questionnaire design tips

Now that you have generated your questions, you should put them together in as attractive and easy to use manner as possible. This will help to maximize your response rate and minimize errors in completion. Here are some useful design tips:

- Give your questionnaire a title that is short and meaningful to the respondent.
- Include clear and concise instructions on how to complete the questionnaire.
- State clearly what the purpose of the research is and who is carrying out the research.
- If your questionnaire contains sensitive items be sure to clearly state your policy on confidentiality. A questionnaire should be valid; it should measure what it is supposed to measure. One of the main threats to validity in a questionnaire survey is the possibility of non-truthful responses to sensitive questions.
- Use short sentences and simple, direct language throughout. Avoid abbreviations. Make sure the reading level required is appropriate for your respondents.
- Begin with non-threatening and interesting items. If the first items are too threatening or 'boring', there is little chance that the person will complete the questionnaire.
- Place the most important items in the first half of the questionnaire as respondents often send back partially completed questionnaires.
- Emphasize crucial words in each item by using bold, italics or underlining.
- Leave adequate space for respondents to provide responses if you are using open questions.
- Vary the question format: respondents tend to lose attention and produce repetitive responses if they lose interest in the questionnaire.
- Group questions into coherent categories. It is disconcerting for respondents if questions jump from topic to topic.
- Use professional production methods to maximize the impression that the questionnaire is important and worth completing.
- End the questionnaire in a gentle and friendly manner, expressing gratitude for the respondent's time and effort.
- Print the return address on the questionnaire itself (because questionnaires often become separated from the reply envelopes). Make returning the questionnaire as easy as possible (for example provide reply-paid envelopes).

Pre-testing

The final test of a questionnaire is to try it on representatives of the target audience. If there are problems with the questionnaire, they almost always show up here. If possible, be present while a respondent is completing the questionnaire and tell him or her that it is OK to ask you for clarification of any item. The questions he or she asks are indicative of problems in the questionnaire (the questions on the questionnaire must be without any ambiguity because there will be no chance to clarify a question when the survey is mailed).

Summary

In designing a questionnaire that is reliable, valid and acceptable to respondents, great care must be taken over wording, response formats and the order of items. Differences in wording can produce very different responses. Questions can be about demographic facts (age, gender, number of children), knowledge, behaviour or attitudes, and the researcher must consider whether the item is an appropriate indicator for the kind of information sought. A key consideration is the target population, and the instrument designed must be pretested with members of the target population before the survey.

Reference

Streiner DL and Norman GR (2003) *Health Measurement Scales: A Practical Guide to Their Development and Use* (3rd edn). Oxford: Oxford University Press.

Further reading

Bowling A (1997) *Measuring Health: A Review of Quality of Life Measurement Scales* (2nd edn.) Milton Keynes: Open University Press.

Quality of life scales are a particular kind of questionnaire that have been developed to measure patient-based outcomes of health care. Bowling's book is an excellent introduction to their use.

12 Survey design

John Browne

Overview

Developing an instrument to use is only part of the task of quantitative research design. This chapter considers the design of the survey, including sampling (deciding who to include), different data-collection methods, and how to improve response rates.

Learning objectives

After working through this chapter you will be better able to:

- **assess the strengths and weaknesses of different sampling strategies**
- **identify ways of making surveys more representative**

Key terms

Generalizability The extent to which the results from a sample survey can be applied to the whole population.

Non-sampling error The amount of error in the data we have collected that is due to problems with the reliability and validity of our data-collection instrument (as opposed to problems with our sampling of the population).

Probability sample Each member of the population has a random and equal chance of being selected.

Response rate The proportion of those sampled who responded.

Sample A group of respondents drawn from a population to represent the whole.

Sampling error Limitations on how far inferences from a sample can be generalized to the whole population.

Purposes of surveys

In Chapters 3 and 4, the importance of specifying a research question and identifying an appropriate method for investigating it was discussed. Research questions in survey work are likely to be mainly descriptive. Surveys are a widely used method for answering such questions as:

- How many rural villagers have access to vaccination programmes?

- How satisfied are patients with their hospital services?
- Are young people more likely to smoke if their parents smoke?
- Which sections of the population are lacking in knowledge about HIV infection risks?

Surveys also aid explanation by generating hypotheses, and analysis may also be used not only to test hypotheses but also to expose interesting *associations*. If we want to demonstrate *causality* (for instance that certain lifestyles *cause* a difference in health status) these associations must be investigated either (a) under more controlled conditions such as an experiment or (b) by a cohort design, in which the same respondents are followed up over time so that the researcher can investigate which variables caused later effects. Cohort designs present particular difficulties for survey management. In this chapter, only the design of single (sometimes called 'snapshot') surveys is considered.

Collecting data

The general term 'survey' covers any research design in which the same variables are measured across a sample of subjects. The subjects can be individuals, households, health care settings or any other unit. This produces a standard set of data for each subject, which can be analysed statistically to look for patterns within the data, regularities and relationships between the variables measured.

There is a range of ways of collecting measurements in surveys. Some rely purely on observation. If the researcher is interested in how many children cycle to school in various parts of the country, one possible data-collection method is to simply count the number of children arriving at the school gates on a bicycle. However, in social science most methods of data collection rely on asking people to report their behaviour, or views, or knowledge. Some of the major methods of data collection are described in Table 12.1, with their advantages and disadvantages. Important considerations are cost, response rate, literacy of the respondents, interviewer bias, whether it is important to probe answers or not, and the need for confidentiality.

Table 12.1 Advantages and disadvantages of different survey methods

Survey method	Advantages	Disadvantages
Personal (face-to-face) interviews	Longer interaction with interviewee possible. More flexibility (e.g. opportunity to probe inconsistent or ambiguous responses).	More costly. Takes longer to carry out. Possibility of interviewer bias. Possibility that interviewees will be less honest about sensitive issues.
Telephone surveys	Faster. Less costly.	Less flexible, especially if using automated dialling survey. Calling time is limited to a window of 6 p.m. to 9 p.m. if representative samples are sought for most surveys: may inconvenience the interviewee.

(Table continued)

Table 12.1 *continued*

Survey method	Advantages	Disadvantages
Telephone surveys	Many aspects of analysis can be performed immediately if using automated dialling systems. Respondents may be more honest about sensitive issues.	Can lead to unrepresentative samples if random dialling is used. Respondents may be less honest if there are people listening.
Mail surveys	Less costly. Allow respondent to answer at leisure. Eliminate interviewer bias. Respondents may be more honest about sensitive issues.	Take longer to carry out. Response rates may be low in populations with lower educational and literacy levels. Less control over how the respondent completes the questionnaire (e.g. they may skip questions). Higher costs. Interviewer bias is less of a problem.
Email surveys	Less costly. Fast to perform. Eliminates interviewer bias. Respondents may be more honest about sensitive issues.	High resistance to 'spam' means an email survey is only useful with people who have agreed to be contacted by email for surveys. People with email not representative of general population.
Internet/intranet surveys	Less costly. Fast to perform and analyse. Can use features (e.g. question skipping logic) not available to paper-based questionnaires. Can be more colourful and attractive to complete. Eliminates interviewer bias. Respondents may be more honest about sensitive issues.	People with Internet not representative of general population. Internet use perceived as more 'casual' and optional: interviewees more likely to quit in the middle of a questionnaire.

How to select the people to be surveyed

Whatever the research question and however the data are to be collected, a key concern is the *generalizability* of a survey. The user of survey results needs to know how far the findings are applicable not only to those surveyed but to the whole population of interest, whether that is all the citizens of a country, all adolescents, or all potential hospital patients. An obvious way of ensuring that the results of an investigation are completely generalizable is to survey the whole population. Occasionally such an exercise is undertaken, as when a population census is undertaken. But such attempts are unwieldy and expensive and so are conducted infrequently. A *sample survey*, if the sample is representative, provides a quicker, more cost-effective, labour-saving way of collecting information about the total population. Results from a smaller sample survey are less unwieldy, and therefore easier to analyse. However, if only a sample is chosen, the researcher needs to consider how representative the respondents are of the whole population. The first task in this process is to clearly define the target population. Obviously, we cannot know if a sample is representative of the population if we don't know what the population looks like.

Sampling methods are classified as either *probability* or *non-probability*. In probability samples, each member of the population has a known probability of being selected. Probability methods include random sampling, systematic sampling and stratified sampling. In non-probability sampling, members are selected from the population in some non-random manner. These include convenience sampling, judgment sampling, quota sampling, and snowball sampling. The advantage of probability sampling is that *sampling error* can be calculated. Sampling error is the degree to which a sample might differ from the population. When inferring to the population, results are reported plus or minus the sampling error. In non-probability sampling, the degree to which the sample differs from the population remains unknown.

Probability sampling

Random sampling is the purest form of probability sampling. Each member of the population has an equal and known chance of being selected. A random sample has to be drawn from a record of the population as a whole, known as a *sampling frame*. If the sample is to be free from bias, the sampling frame should be as complete a record as possible of the total population. Typical sampling frames include registers of patients in primary health care, electoral roll registers, and postcode address files. It quickly becomes clear that such options are more of a reality in highly developed countries than in those that are less well developed and where records are likely to be less complete. Even in countries in which such sources of data are available, in practice no records are perfect, and a trade-off still has to be made between the advantages and disadvantages of each potential data source. All of these contain their own characteristic bias. Electoral registers, for instance, neglect the homeless, the highly mobile, and those who fail to complete forms.

Systematic sampling is often used instead of random sampling. After the required sample size has been calculated, every Nth record is selected from a list of population members. As long as the list does not contain any hidden order, this sampling method is in practice often as good as the random sampling method, although we do need to be aware that there may be 'hidden' biases in ordering of lists such as those of surnames. The advantage of the systematic over the random sampling technique is simplicity. Systematic sampling is frequently used to select a specified number of records from a computer file.

Stratified sampling is a commonly used probability method that is superior to random sampling because it reduces sampling error. A *stratum* is a subset of the population whose members share at least one common characteristic. The researcher first identifies the relevant strata and their actual representation in the population. Random sampling is then used to select subjects from each stratum until the number of subjects in that stratum is proportional to its frequency in the population. Stratified sampling is often used when one or more of the strata in the population have a low incidence relative to the other stratums.

Cluster sampling assumes that populations are built up of relevant hierarchies of sampling units. For instance, individuals belong to households, which are clustered in small areas, and then into larger ones. Nurses could be contacted as individuals, or as part of a ward, or of a hospital. Cluster sampling is the sampling of complete groups of units, such as all the households in an area, or all the nurses on a series of wards. Cluster sampling methods offer convenience and often cost savings. It is, for instance, easier to carry out fieldwork for a household survey if covering all households in particular clusters than contacting a random sample of individual households spread over a whole country. The disadvantage is that they increase sampling error.

✎ Activity 12.1

Consider possible sources of bias that might affect the following studies, and the implications for the studies in each case:

1 A postal questionnaire administered to a random sample drawn from a primary health care register of patients.
2 A telephone survey of young people, using a random sample drawn from a telephone directory.

↻ Feedback

1 Registers of patients are often inaccurate. Patients may not inform staff of new addresses, so the survey will under-report those who are mobile. Those with no fixed address have little chance of inclusion. If the target population had a low literacy rate, this would also reduce the representativeness of any self-completed questionnaire.

2 As the telephone directory will not list age, a screening question is needed to identify target respondents. There may be biases in adults' willingness to provide information about resident young people. Any telephone survey will be biased towards those who are wealthier and more likely to own a telephone. Also, the interviewer may not know whether the respondent is in a room with other people which may inhibit open responses.

How large should a probability sample be?

In general, the larger the sample the more closely it will approximate to the characteristics of the global population from which it was drawn, and the greater the likelihood that the results will be statistically significant. A survey should not be dismissed as unreliable simply because the sample size is small. A relatively modest sample may be large enough to satisfy the aims of the study. The research question is all-important. Obviously cost and time resources are important considerations when choosing a sample size. The following are also important.

Prevalence of target event/behaviour

If your survey is intended to detect something rare then one is likely to need a large sample. Supposing 2% of a population have attended a sexually transmitted disease (STD) clinic in the last year. A sample of 10,000 will yield only 200 individuals who report having attended an STD clinic. If we want to know more about these people (such as their gender and age) we quickly run into trouble. Analysis by gender would reduce this number by half for each sex, and further analysis by age group might result in only 25 in the subgroup of women aged 16–25.

Variation in target event/behaviour

Sometimes we are interested in variables that cannot be simply described in yes/no format. Take, for example, a study that includes measurement of how often women visit a family planning service. The majority may be clustered in the middle of the distribution, making one or two visits a year; there may be a further proportion who have made such a visit only once in the past year and there may be another, equally rare, subgroup who have visited more than times in a year. If an aim of the survey is to measure a range of behaviours or events then it must be large enough to capture these extremes.

Activity 12.2

Rare or diverse behaviours and characteristics can be studied by drawing a random sample from the population, when there is no more appropriate sampling frame. However, to find enough cases for analysis, the sample has to be very large and wastefully collect data about people who are not of interest. Can you think of any alternative sampling strategies for identifying relatively uncommon behaviours? Think about the problems posed by the following two research questions and suggest how a sample could be identified for a survey.

1 How often do injecting drug users share needles?
2 Do urban homeless people have access to primary care services?

Feedback

1 Drug use is illegal in many societies, and those who inject drugs are unlikely to be listed on any 'official' records which could be used as a sampling frame. A whole population sample may well underestimate numbers, as drug users may be less willing to complete survey questionnaires. Instead, it may be possible to survey users of a relevant clinic, if there is one, by asking patients attending to complete a questionnaire.

2 Any survey that aims to assess 'unmet need' (those not receiving a service who could benefit) clearly cannot use a register of current service users as a sampling frame. As the homeless are difficult to identify through records, any survey would have to use methods of recruiting respondents where they were, perhaps on the streets or in facilities provided for use by homeless people.

Non-probability sampling

Any sample that is not drawn randomly from a known population is called a non-probability sample. As the two examples above illustrate, there are situations in which it is preferable to use non-probability sampling, although the disadvantage is that it is impossible to know how representative the survey sample is. Some common methods of non-probability samples are described below.

Purposive sampling involves the deliberate choice of respondents, subjects, or settings to reflect some features or characteristics of interest, for example patients with terminal cancer.

Convenience sampling is where samples are selected because they are conveniently available. This non-probability method is often used during preliminary research efforts to obtain a rough estimate of the results, without incurring the cost or taking the time required to select a random sample.

Snowball samples are collected by networking out from a convenience or purposive sample to reach more covert or inaccessible subjects. Respondents might be asked to introduce the researcher to others who meet the sample criteria. While this technique can dramatically lower search costs, it comes at the expense of introducing bias because the technique itself reduces the likelihood that the sample will represent a good cross section from the population.

Quota samples are allocated according to proportional distribution of different demographic characteristics, such as gender, age, region, social class. The quota sample has the advantage of being representative in terms of known characteristics, but not necessarily of others, because there is no way of knowing what the response rate is. For example if the age distribution of a population is such that 40% are under age 25, 35% are aged 25 to 40 and 25% are aged over 40, then the quota sample would be drawn up to represent exactly these proportions.

All these non-probability samples present the typical limitations of volunteer samples, that is they are likely to contain bias related to the variable under study. Suppose the focus of investigation was on health-seeking behaviour relating to stress. The most stressed members of the population might be least likely to agree to take part because of pressure of time.

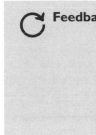

Activity 12.3

Make a note of possible biases the following situations might present if used in a quota sample survey, and the implications for the study.

1 Administering questionnaires at a mainline railway station in the morning to investigate knowledge of local health care facilities.
2 Carrying out a face-to-face interview with shoppers outside a supermarket during a weekday afternoon to investigate use of alternative health care in one city.

Feedback

1 The sample would be biased towards those who travel in the morning, who are more likely to be in well-paid jobs. At a mainline station there are also likely to be many respondents from outside the area who would not know about local health care services.

2 This strategy would predominantly identify people with no full-time paid work, and would not be generalizable to the whole population.

How can we tell if the sample is representative or not?

Even when samples are drawn randomly from a reliable sampling frame, the researcher still needs to consider the representativeness of the final sample (those who agreed to take part). There are two main techniques for maximizing representativeness: improving the response rate, and comparing the sample and the population.

Improving the response rate

All samples are volunteer samples at the point of contact because people cannot be coerced into taking part, hence the importance of the response rate to a random sample. The higher it is, the greater the confidence with which results can be generalized to the population as a whole. Typical response rates for government-instigated surveys tend to be around 80%; for other surveys the response rate may be more typically 60% to 70%. Response rates lower than 60% would raise concern relating to bias in the sample, and throw into question the generalizability of the findings. A high response rate gives a good guarantee that there will be little response bias, while a low response rate gives more cause for concern. We cannot know a great deal about those who do not agree to take part, by definition, because if they are not prepared to answer the questions relating to the investigation they are unlikely to answer questions relating to why they did not.

Activity 12.4

Think of some ways in which you could maximize the response rate to:

1   A postal questionnaire survey of health professionals in your country
2   A face-to-face interview survey of nurses in one hospital.

Feedback

1   Possible ways to improve response rates might include:

   • a letter persuading respondents that the survey was worthwhile
   • reminder letters for those who did not reply
   • assurances of confidentiality
   • use of a well written and designed questionnaire.

2   In a face-to-face interview, the calibre of the interviewer is crucial. He or she must be trained to provide information about the study, answer any questions and reassure the respondents that their views will remain confidential. It might be better to use interviewers who are from outside the hospital. Again, information about the need for the research, or how it might be of benefit for the respondents, might help.

In some surveys, respondents are rewarded in some way for taking part. This is more common in commercial settings than in health care research, but in some surveys it might be worth considering payment, in cash or as goods. The disadvantage (apart from increasing the costs of the survey) is that if it is known that the researcher will be paying for respondents there is then a potential bias towards those who need the reward most.

Many factors, then, may influence the response rate. If the survey is being carried out by a research team with a good reputation, from a credible institution, and if the research questions being asked are important and serious, then respondents are more likely to feel favourably inclined towards taking part in it.

Comparing the sample and the population

The second way of ensuring that a sample is representative is to compare the structure of the achieved sample and the structure of the global population it represents. You can find out whether the survey was representative in terms of known variables. These are likely to be demographic information. In most countries, data are collected in censuses on age, gender, educational level, social class and area of residence. The profile of the achieved sample can be compared with the demographic profile of the population it represents to see how well it 'behaves'. Of course, you can never know how typical the sample was in terms of other variables. People who do not take part are likely to be different from those who do in ways that can be important to the integrity of the study. Some researchers have reported that people who respond to surveys answer questions differently from those who do not. Others have found that late responders answer differently from early responders and that the differences may be due to the different levels of interest in the subject matter. Demographic characteristics of non-respondents have also been investigated by many researchers. Non-response is sometimes associated with low education. In some surveys it will be possible to compare to some extent the characteristics of non-responders, if we have some information from the sampling frame about them. This could help in identifying particular kinds of bias.

Limitations of survey designs

In Chapter 10, it was noted that quantitative social science had its roots in the development of 'social statistics' in northern Europe. Although the governments of all countries now use extensive 'fact gathering' about their populations, the acceptability of interviewing and form filling is not universal. Self-completion questionnaires obviously rely on relatively high levels of literacy. In many societies, the notion of an interview itself might be alien, and in others it might be quite threatening. Where, for instance, 'state surveillance' is used to control sections of the population, citizens may be justifiably suspicious of the uses to which survey findings will be put. There may also be a desire on the part of survey respondents to 'tell the interviewer what they want to hear'. This is similar to the 'social desirability' or 'courtesy' bias we discussed in Chapter 11.

For example, one anthropological study using qualitative methods uncovered the severe limitations of previous surveys (Stone and Campbell 1984). The researchers found that cultural traditions and unfamiliarity with questionnaires had led Nepalese villagers to feign ignorance of abortion and family planning services and to under-report their use of contraception and abortion when responding to surveys. These problems are often termed 'non-sampling error', which we shall discuss below.

Sampling error and non-sampling error

So far in this chapter we have only discussed sampling error, which is error due to selecting a sample that is not representative of the population as whole. *Sampling error* can occur for a number of reasons, including too small a sample size or because we used invalid sampling methods (for example, sampling only people with access to the Internet when trying to make inferences about the general population). Crucially, sampling error is something that, in theory, we can identify and control.

Non-sampling error is a more profound challenge to the survey design because it introduces biases that undermine the reliability and validity of our findings. Non-sampling error occurs because of problems with our data-collection instrument. These problems may be due to poor reliability (too much random noise in our instrument) or poor validity (the instrument systematically 'misses' what it is supposed to measure). One of the main non-sampling errors referred to by Stone and Campbell (1984) is a problem of validity: the survey instruments are influenced heavily by 'courtesy bias' (the tendency to tell the interviewer what the respondent thinks they want to hear), causing the instrument to systematically miss the concept targeted (such as the 'true' awareness and use of contraceptive devices in Nepal).

How could we have detected this non-sampling error? Qualitative work provides detailed descriptions of cultural values, which could have been used to design questions that were appropriate and to inform researchers of the cultural context. Ethnographic research can be used for 'triangulation' to validate the findings of survey research.

However, it should also be noted that this unduly privileges findings from ethnographic work, which are then seen as the 'gold standard' of truth. Stone and Campbell suggest that survey research and more traditional anthropological methods badly need to be guided and supplemented by one another if social science research is genuinely to assist development planning in non-industrialized countries.

Summary

Designing a survey involves deciding how to collect the data needed and who to sample to answer the research question. Probability samples should be representative of the whole population, but it may not be possible to achieve this. Non-probability designs may be necessary to identify rare behaviours or hard-to-reach subjects. Whatever the sampling strategy, attention must be paid to how representative the sample is in order to improve the generalizability of the survey.

Surveys are an invaluable method for accessing standardized information across a sample of the population. However, to provide valid and meaningful results they are best used in conjunction with qualitative methods which can aid the development of an appropriate instrument and provide information about the context of findings. Using surveys may present particular problems in developing countries.

References

Stone L and Campbell JG (1984) The use and misuse of surveys in international development: an experiment from Nepal. *Human Organisation* 43(1): 27–37.

Further reading

De Vaus, DA, (2002) *Surveys in Social Research*. London: Routledge.

This is a good example of the number of general books about social research design on the market, which all deal with issues of sampling, design and organisation.

http://www.caps.ucfs.edu/capsweb/projects/c&tindex.html

This is just one example of a Web site that publishes questionnaires and manuals for training survey interviewers. This particular example is for a survey of counselling and HIV testing in East Africa, but a little searching should identify other sites for projects. These can be an invaluable source of information about how other researchers have designed questionnaires, and of example questionnaires that can sometimes be used as models for your own instruments.

Nyandieka LN, Bowden A, Wanjau J and Fox-Rushby JA (2002) How to do (or not to do) . . . managing a household survey: a practical example from the KENQOL survey. *Health Policy and Planning* 17: 207–12.

This is a useful case study from Kenya on some of the practical issues that have to be dealt with in planning a successful survey on health related quality of life.

Practical: designing a questionnaire

John Browne

Overview

This practical chapter gives you an opportunity to design your own short questionnaire, which could be used in a survey.

Learning objectives

After working through this chapter you will be better able to

- **relate what you have learned about questionnaires and surveys to your own practical experience.**

Introduction

To complete the chapter to the stage where the questionnaire is finalized, you will need:

- any notes you made for Chapter 9, when you carried out a qualitative analysis on your chosen topic
- to review Chapter 11 on the design of questionnaires
- to make about five copies of the questionnaire for use in piloting
- five members of the target population who will agree to help you pilot the questionnaire

✏ Activity 13.1

The qualitative data you produced in Chapter 9 may well have generated some quantitative research questions on the topic you chose. Frame one of these as a question, which could be answered using a survey design. If your data did not raise any appropriate questions, the following are some suggestions for research questions that you might refine for this practical chapter.

1 How does patient satisfaction with health care delivery vary between different patient groups? Restrict your question to one health care setting (for example, a primary care centre or one outpatient department) and choose two groups to sample, such as men and women, or patients with different conditions.

2 How well do professionals understand the roles of other professional groups within your health care organization? Think about aspects of the role of one group that

might be uncertain, such as perceptions of what tasks a practice nurse might carry out, or what clinicians' attitude to the role of the hospital administrative staff might be.

3 What proportion of nurses (or people in the community) report using infection control procedures (such as appropriate hand washing)? You might want to consider an infection control policy in force within your organization (if there is one) and whether your respondents are aware of it, or its contents.

Use the notes below to guide you in planning, preparing and piloting your questionnaire. If time permits and you wish to do so, you may then choose to carry out a mini-survey using the questionnaire you have designed.

Guidance notes

When you have framed a research question, decide which population you are interested in (doctors in your hospital, patients of a clinic, all the people who live within the district covered by your health agency). How would you select a representative sample of this population? Would a convenience, or other non-probability, sample be adequate for your needs?

Next, think about relevant indicators for the variables you are interested in. Construct a short questionnaire (with no more than 12 items), designed for self-completion, containing items that collect some of the following kinds of data:

- demographic information (such as gender, age)
- knowledge
- attitudes
- reports of behaviour.

Check that each item you choose for inclusion has all the desirable characteristics discussed in Chapter 11:

- neutral wording
- avoids asking two or more questions at the same time
- accommodates all possible answers
- has mutually exclusive response choices, so that a single answer cannot fall into more than one category
- unambiguous differences between the response choices
- produces variability of responses
- does not make unwarranted assumptions
- does not ask questions where the respondent has to guess (satisfice) the correct answer
- does not imply a desired answer

For each item, choose how respondents will answer.

Will there be a pre-defined response set? If so, think through all possible responses so that there is an appropriate response for every respondent. If not, you need to think about how you will code responses.

If you are asking respondents to agree or disagree with statements to indicate their attitudes, how many responses do you need? Do you need a 'neutral' category?

If you are looking at reported behaviour, think about how to phrase questions so that they minimize recall and other sources of bias. For instance, asking 'How often did you visit the doctor this month?' may lead to more accurate reporting than asking about 'an average year'. However, you must also take account of the likely frequency of events. In a general population survey, for instance, most people will not have visited the doctor at all in one month.

Also think carefully about phrasing questions about sensitive issues such as sexual behaviour. You need to consider what is 'sensitive' in your setting, as this is culturally specific. In Britain, some women consider 'age' to be sensitive information, for instance.

Next try and design your questionnaire in as attractive and comprehensible a fashion as possible. Check that you have met all the design tips mentioned in Chapter 12:

- short, meaningful title
- clear and concise instructions
- clear statement of purpose, identifying who is carrying out the survey
- clear statement of policy on confidentiality
- simple, direct language throughout
- begin with non-threatening and interesting items
- place the most important items in the first half of the questionnaire
- emphasize crucial words in each item by using bold, italics or underlining
- leave adequate space for respondents to provide responses
- vary the question format
- group questions into coherent categories.
- use professional production methods
- end the questionnaire in a gentle and friendly manner
- print the return address on the questionnaire itself.

Finally, consider how you are going to distribute and collect your questionnaire and, if you are not going to introduce it in person, what kind of introduction and explanation you will enclose with it.

Phrasing good questions for a survey is a more difficult task than it appears. A question whose meaning seems obvious to you might confuse your colleagues, and some respondents may be offended by a question that appears innocuous to others. There may be valid responses to a question that did not occur to you. This is why you need to pilot your instrument.

Piloting

Give your questionnaire to at least five respondents (choose people from the population your questionnaire is aimed at). Ask them to go through it and give you feedback on how easy it was to complete and whether there were any questions that were difficult or insensitive. Check that they understood questions in the way you intended. If not, how could you improve the wording?

Was the layout clear and inviting, or was it difficult for them to see where they should make their response? Use the feedback from the piloting exercise to review and amend your questionnaire.

Activity 13.2

Survey (optional)

After making any necessary amendments, you can use your questionnaire in a mini-survey if time permits. The sample size needed to produce statistically significant findings (that is, findings that we can be confident are not just due to chance) about relationships between variables will depend on your question and the likely variation in the population. However, if you are just interested in descriptive frequencies (such as how many people have a particular attitude or how often they have experienced a particular event) try to hand out 30 questionnaires.

Reflection

1 If your response rate was low, how could it be improved?
2 Were there questions which did not discriminate well between your respondents? For instance, if everyone agrees that 'good health care is a priority', this is not really worth asking.
3 Were there any items that were often left blank? Why might this be?
4 What, if any, are the implications for policy or practice in your results?
5 If you were to survey a larger sample, how could you test the reliability of your questionnaire?
6 What kinds of validity would it be important to test?

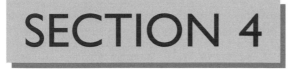

SECTION 4

Social science disciplines in public health

14 Introduction to applied medical anthropology

Karina Kielmann

Overview

This chapter introduces concepts and methodological approaches underlying the application of medical anthropology in public health. Consideration of the current role of applied medical anthropology in public health is followed by a discussion of focal areas, methodological approaches and ethical concerns in the anthropological investigation of health and health-seeking behaviour.

Learning objectives

After working through this chapter, you will be able to:

- describe the core concepts in medical anthropology
- conduct a simple illness narrative for gathering information on illness explanatory models
- understand the choice of more or less structured methods in applied medical anthropology
- describe the ethical issues in conducting anthropological work in health settings

Key terms

Explanatory model Systematic set of knowledge, beliefs and attitudes with regard to a particular illness which offers explanations of illness and treatment to guide choices among available therapies and to cast personal and social meaning on the experience of illness.

Illness behaviour The way a person behaves when they feel a need for better health.

Medical pluralism The existence of more than one medical tradition. Nearly all societies are medically pluralistic.

Medical sectors Components that make up the medical system, usually including a *popular* sector (lay, non-professional), a *folk* sector (non-professional, specialist) and *professional* sectors (organized, institutionalized) (Kleinman 1981).

Medical systems Sets of premises and ideas that enable people to organize their perceptions and experiences of medical events (such as illness episodes) and to organize their interventions for affecting and controlling these events.

Medical traditions Distinctive combination of ideas, practices, skills, tools and materials that are related to recognizing, explaining and treating illness conditions.

Patterns of resort The paths people make as they pick and choose their ways from one sector of the medical system to another, in search of diagnosis, treatment and other services.

Therapy management group The set of individuals involved in diagnosing cause and consequence of affliction, making choices about the therapeutic options to adopt and directing the course of therapy.

Medical anthropology in international public health

What is medical anthropology?

Medical anthropology is a subfield of cultural anthropology and examines how people in different societies explain the causes of illness and go about seeking treatment. It situates patterns of health and illness as well as health perceptions and health-seeking behaviour within a wider ecological, social, political and economic context. The field is divided into a number of theoretical streams (for example, ecological, politico-economic, symbolic, feminist) that differ according to their analytical focus in the study of health and illness. Applied medical anthro-pology is not a separate theoretical stream but one that generally refers to the application of anthropological methods in public health and health systems research.

Generally, applied medical anthropology takes place in collaboration with public health scientists within a setting that usually involves a 'donor' agency and a 'recipient' population, whereby actors can be agencies, practitioners, communities and so forth. The assumption is that anthropologists, because of a uniquely humanist and interpretive approach, can best discern what the recipient com-munity knows, believes, understands, needs, wants and does in terms of health. Goals of the collaboration are fairly instrumental and tied to public health outcomes. Specifically, anthropologists have been hired to:

- assist in culturally appropriate design, implementation and evaluation of health interventions
- elucidate why health interventions are adopted or rejected
- examine the interaction between providers and patients
- communicate public health messages in a culturally sensitive manner.

Anthropological approaches and health-related areas of interest

What makes the anthropological approach distinctive?

Anthropology means the science of man, or humankind. It is a *humanistic* discipline, in other words, deeply concerned with humans and their lives. Anthropologists are interested in understanding the personal, the subjective and the experiential basis of knowledge and practice rather than abstract, general and representative observations. In exploring subjectivity of human experience, anthropologists tend to espouse some degree of *cultural relativism* to their observations, suggesting that 'cultures' are coherent, systematic and rational within their own context. Situating individual elements of a 'culture' in a particular *context* (social, historical, political) is important for any *interpretation*, that is, the anthropologist's attempt to understand the deeper, underlying meanings that guide how people think, act, interact, how and why they modify the material and social environments they live in.

Why is health of interest to an anthropologist?

Anthropologists see health, illness and the process of healing as cultural phenomena that can be analysed ('made sense of') within specific sociocultural settings. Biomedicine is understood as only one of many medical systems in the world, and medical systems themselves can be analysed as cultural systems of knowledge and practice. This seems counterintuitive: it is difficult to think of health and illness as cultural 'events' when they are so obviously connected with bodily experience, and thus paradigmatically biological. The following activity prompts you to reflect on how illness episodes are socially and culturally embedded:

Activity 14.1

Recall the last time you had a common cold. Read the questions below and jot down what you can recall in the order of the questions, so that you have a sequential *illness narrative* that describes your experience, perceptions of, and response to the cold. If you haven't experienced one, ask a family member or friend.

1 What told you something was wrong?
2 What was the first thing you did? Who was the first person you spoke to about it?
3 What happened then?
4 What was the next thing you did?
5 Why do you think this happened?

Feedback

The answers you gave could be listed as in Table 14.1. 'Patterns of resort' are the ways in which people seek treatment or relief for their symptoms. The answer to 'Why do you think this happened?' is your perceived aetiology.

Table 14.1 Example of a recorded illness narrative

Perceived symptoms	Had scratchy throat, pain in ears. Felt tired and achy.
First pattern of resort	Gargled with hot salt water, had Lemsip, went to bed early. Called my dad.
Perceived outcome 1	Felt worse the next day. Sore throat, difficulty in swallowing.
Second pattern of resort	Stayed in bed. Had tea with honey. Eventually took some antibiotics (left over from last chest infection).
Perceived aetiology	Long-distance travel on a plane (air-conditioning and people coughing a lot). Also overworked and a lot of stress in the preceding weeks.

The method you used to elicit information about the illness experience produces an *illness narrative*. This generally covers perceived symptomatology, patterns of resort (those ways in which people navigate their way through the popular, folk and professional sectors of the medical system in search of treatment and relief), perceived course of illness, perceived aetiology and perceived outcome. If you had collected a hundred illness narratives for the 'common cold' and organized the information in a systematic way, you would be able to develop an *explanatory model* of the common cold. Investigating local explanatory models of illness is very much at the heart of applied medical anthropology and is based in an approach developed by the anthropologist-physician Arthur Kleinman in the early 1980s. The idea of an explanatory model is linked to a central distinction that medical anthropologists make between *disease* and *illness*. While a biomedical definition of disease is largely based on demonstrable physical changes in the body's structure or function that can be quantified by reference to 'normal' physiological measurements, illness is the subjective evaluation or response of a patient to his or her feeling unwell. It includes experience but also the meanings given to that experience.

Given that we would expect much agreement across the narratives in terms of what signs constitute a common cold, what commonly accepted home remedies are, at what point one conventionally seeks treatment outside the home, and so forth, collecting 100 narratives on the common cold might not seem a terribly exciting or surprising exercise in a familiar setting. However, the important point that anthropologists try to make is that what we take for granted as 'common sense' is far from common sense, but the product of our socialization in a particular sociocultural context that values or privileges particular types of knowledge as legitimate and authoritative. So the exercise here is to ask questions about what we hold as common-sense, shared, authoritative knowledge on different dimensions of illness. The type of 'data' collected in an illness narrative points to four key areas and questions for research for applied medical anthropologists, which are listed in Table 14.2.

✎ Activity 14.2

Use the questions listed in Table 14.2 to reflect critically on the illness narrative data you recorded for Activity 14.1. To what extent are the 'data' context bound?

Table 14.2 Key areas and questions in applied medical anthropology

Key area	General questions	Example: the 'common cold'
Perceptions of health and illness	How is illness defined and recognized? How do people evaluate severity of an illness? At what point are signs of being unwell legitimately 'translated' into symptoms of illness? How does the language used to talk about illness reflect social reality of a particular setting?	Where does the label 'common cold' come from? What signs and symptoms delimit the 'common cold'? At what point is a 'cold' deemed serious? What do perceived causes of the 'cold' reflect in terms of how we understand the relationship between the mind, body, society and the environment?
Health-seeking or illness behaviour	What are societal responses and implications of illness? When, where and how is relief from illness sought? What constitute appropriate or legitimate treatment options for particular ailments?	Which people are considered legitimate sources of advice when you have a 'cold' and why? At what point is a 'cold' serious enough to seek help outside lay sources? What differentiates lay and professional remedies for a 'cold' and where do you obtain them?
Medical systems	What options for care/relief exist? How are they organized and ranked in terms of access, acceptability, and authority?	What/who determines your sequential pattern of care seeking?
Healing and therapeutic efficacy	How is health restored? To what extent do therapeutic actions produce expected outcomes? What does efficacy mean locally?	What makes you feel better when you have a 'cold'? Why?

↻ Feedback

Reflecting on narratives of the 'common cold' might include the following: cultural specificity and legitimacy around the symptom 'cluster' and body parts associated with a 'cold', folk aetiologies of the 'cold' (such as preoccupation with the relationship between stress and immunity, theories of contagion); acceptability of certain home and over-the-counter remedies; points at which the 'sick role' becomes socially acceptable; perceived turning points that invoke particular care-seeking decisions.

We see here that the labels given to illnesses, the thresholds at which illness behaviour is initiated, and the perceived legitimacy and efficacy of particular treatment options are grounded in the wider social context of a *medical belief system* that is less an institutional structure than a set of ideas that guide people's response to illness episodes. Nearly all medical systems are pluralistic, in that they comprise multiple, sometimes conflicting, *medical traditions*. These traditions have more or less institutional and social legitimacy according to their location in professional, folk and lay or popular *medical sectors*.

Activity 14.3

Try listing all the medical traditions that exist in the country that you reside and group them according to their location in the popular (lay), folk or professional sectors. Where are the divisions between sectors clear, and where are they less clear (for example, where might they overlap)?

Feedback

In listing the medical traditions that exist in the area you live in, you may have found it harder to think where to place traditions that may be institutionalized in some form, but have mixed recognition and social legitimacy, because they are considered 'alternative', 'complementary', 'traditional' and so forth (for example, homeopathy) Likewise, it may be difficult to categorize folk practitioners who have recently become professionalized (such as trained 'traditional' birth attendants).

Most treatment seeking is initiated within the non-professional sector, in what Janzen (1978) first described as *therapy management groups*. These are those individuals involved in diagnosing the causes and consequences of afflictions and making choices about how to choose between therapeutic options. Illness narratives therefore offer insight into people's patterns of resort. The illness narrative is one example of a semi-structured method used in applied medical anthropology to better understand people's health perceptions and health-seeking behaviour. In the next section, we review other methods used in this field.

Methodology in medical anthropology

What methodological principles underlie an anthropological approach?

Methodology in anthropology is characterized by flexibility, depth and iteration (repetition over time, for instance by going back to ask interviewees further questions as your research evolves). Traditionally, as anthropologists strive to understand local and *emic* ('insider') perspectives and ways of doing things, they use the most open-ended and unstructured methods possible. For classical anthropologists, who have undergone training in anthropology, this means a mandatory rite of passage of *fieldwork* at one or many points in their life, that is total immersion, *participant observation* and the *holistic* study of a community. The product of long-term fieldwork, called an *ethnography*, does not necessarily have a researcher-driven focal topic but instead comprises a comprehensive study of the interrelationships between environment, economic and social organization, politics, science, religion, medicine, and so forth, in a community.

However, for applied medical anthropologists, many of whom do not necessarily have classical anthropological training, who have a time-bound public health agenda, long-term fieldwork is considered a luxury, and not always necessary for practical application. Most applied anthropologists do not produce ethnographies, but collect data with the help of qualitative guidelines and instruments. These methods can be situated on a continuum from less structured to more structured. By structure, we mean the extent to which a researcher narrows down or predetermines the type of data elicited, for example by asking open-ended or close-ended questions. In a health-related research study, there may be a *triangulation* of methods (the use of more than one method or sources of information to look at a topic) in order to obtain a richer picture and understanding of what is going on. Note that triangulation is often seen as a means of cross-validation of data, however it is equally interesting to consider the discrepancies and differences in perspectives that may be brought to light through a comparison of the data obtained. Triangulation is discussed further in Chapter 16.

Activity 14.4

An anthropologist intending to understand adolescent contraceptive practices might use a number of different methods to better understand perceptions, values, meanings and context of adolescent contraceptive behaviour. These could include focus group discussions with adolescents (community and clinic based), interviews with parents, interviews with family planning providers, records maintained in family planning clinics and an analysis of popular magazines targeted at adolescents. Why would a comparison of these different data sources be useful or interesting?

Feedback

A comparison of the data obtained through these sources might confirm some consistency across the cultural ideals of adolescent behaviour, however it might also reveal underlying conflicts, tensions and points of negotiation between different actors (youth, parents, providers) and discourses (youth culture, public health, popular media, morality norms and so forth).

Qualitative methods used in medical anthropology include:

- observations (direct and indirect)
- interviews (individual and group)
- audio and visual documentation

- analysis of written materials and records
- analysis of drawings and maps.

Table 14.3 indicates different types of observations and interviews that range from very open-ended to highly structured. It is not necessary for you to know what each of these methods is in detail, but rather to think through the factors that would prompt a choice of less or more structured methods (such as subject area, type of setting, purpose of research).

Table 14.3 Examples of methods used in applied medical anthropology

	Less structured →	Semi-structured →	More structured
Observations	Participant observation	Guideline	Spot-checks, checklists
Interviews	Life histories, key informant interviews	Illness narratives, focus group guidelines	KAP survey, ranking exercises

KAP = knowledge, attitudes and practices, a structured questionnaire

Observations are often characterized according to the presence of the researcher (*open* or *hidden*), the extent of his/her *participation* in the event being observed, and whether a phenomenon, such as smoking behaviour, is directly observed (people smoking in a bar) versus indirectly observed (the number of cigarette stubs in ashtrays). Different types of observation may be used in the same study, as illustrated in the following example.

Nutritional anthropologists who want to examine the issue of gender bias in child feeding practices in Community M might spend an initial phase of research observing child care, including feeding practices in households. They may or may not participate directly in household activities. After some time, they might have gained enough understanding of some basic criteria that will enable them to draw up a structured checklist to focus observations around measurable aspects of child feeding practices (such as amount of food, types of food, when meals are taken, and who eats together). Note that the data generated during the initial phase of research not only serve an instrumental purpose to inform the development of a locally valid close-ended tool but provide rich, contextual information that can bring 'life' to the structured data.

Interviews can be conducted with individuals or with groups and can also range from very loosely structured conversations around a basic list of topics to highly structured schedules that are precoded. It is important to note that anthropologists would be unlikely to work with a survey instrument unless they were very familiar with the area and topic, and had perhaps carried out some open-ended, in-depth research beforehand in order to obtain a better sense of the questions and the categories of response that would be relevant to a particular setting.

An anthropologist studying migrant workers' HIV-related risk perceptions and behaviours might first conduct a series of migration histories to better understand the context, meaning, and patterns of risks involved in the life trajectories of migrants. After some time, they might be in a better position to conduct a structured ranking exercise, in which migrants are asked to rank a number of risks that they face or are likely to face in order of importance. As in the previous example, interpreting the way in which risks are ranked (structured data) will only make sense if seen in the light of the contextual, narrative data provided through the migration histories.

What do anthropological data look like?

As is probably clear by now, anthropological data tend to be textual and narrative rather than numerical. Data are recorded through extensive note taking or tape recording. To preserve the richness of narrative data, it is often literally transcribed, translated and back-translated to ensure that it is as close to the original utterances as possible. The aim in interpreting textual data is not to isolate individual descriptive elements of interest to the researcher, but rather to look at how they make sense in context. In other words, we try to go beyond the literal, face value of what is said or observed, and attempt to relate what people say and do in relation to their life circumstances and social surroundings.

Ethical issues in anthropological research

Collecting and interpreting anthropological data through fieldwork invoke a number of ethical issues that have been problematized by anthropologists themselves in more recent critical work. These include how open or hidden anthropologists are about their role as researchers, issues concerning how data are shared with subjects of study and – perhaps the most central 'problem' to contemporary anthropology – issues around representation of the 'other' (who has the right to represent, and how?) and resulting concerns about reflexivity (that is, the anthropologist's own positioning in the field and vis-à-vis the subject).

Summary

Medical anthropology's contribution to public health problem solving and research has led to a better understanding of health perceptions and health-seeking behaviour. Anthropologists approach health perceptions, health-seeking behaviour and health systems as cultural phenomena, aiming to situate individual illness experiences in a wider social, cultural and political context. Methods used in applied medical anthropology range from less to more structured, and are characterized by flexibility, depth, iteration and triangulation. The use of anthropological methods in public health raises a number of ethical issues for researchers concerning their role and their access to, and representation of, the subject.

References

Janzen J (1978) *The Quest for Therapy: Medical Pluralism in Lower Zaire*. Berkeley: University of California Press.

Kleinman A (1981) *Patients and Healers in the Context of Culture*. Berkeley: University of California Press.

Young A (1976) Internalizing and externalizing medical belief systems: an Ethiopian example. *Social Science and Medicine* 10: 147–56.

Further reading

Bernard HR (2002) *Research Methods in Anthropology: Qualitative and Quantitative Approaches* (3rd edn). Walnut Creek, CA: AltaMira Press.

This is aimed at students without a disciplinary background in anthropology, and is an excellent practical guide to fieldwork for applied ethnographic research.

Hahn R (ed) (1999) *Anthropology in Public Health: Bridging Differences in Culture and Society.* Oxford: Oxford University Press

This collection of case studies illustrates how anthropology has contributed to public health research and practice.

15 | Introduction to history in health

Virginia Berridge

Overview

This chapter introduces concepts and methodological approaches relevant to the use of historical approaches in public health. A brief section on the role of history in health is followed by a discussion of historical methods, how to use and interpret sources and oral history interviews, and the role of interpretation in history.

Learning objectives

After working through this chapter, you should be able to

- describe concepts in the history of health
- understand the nature of historical methods and how and when they can be used
- understand the role of evidence-based interpretation in history and the nature of competing interpretations

Key terms

Archive A formal location where documentary and visual materials are gathered together and organized. May also refer to a private individual's collection of personal papers, or to an electronic archive, where materials on a topic are available online.

Documentary sources All sources of historical information that are written or printed. They may be verbal or visual.

Historical demography The construction and use of historical data sets to examine issues of mortality, morbidity and fertility.

Historiography The study of what secondary sources say about an historical subject and how this interpretation has changed.

Oral history Interview-based recollection of events in the past.

Presentism A view of historical events that takes its reference point from the present day situation, rather than trying to assess the past on its own terms.

Primary historical sources The materials that historians find and use in their research. These are the evidence on which historians base their arguments.

Secondary historical sources What other historians have written about the past.

Whig history A view of history that assumes the past is a process of inevitable progress to the present.

History in public health

What is history?

History is the past and can cover literally everything. It can range from our national heritage to your personal 'roots'. It means literally a story, an oral or written record of the past, or the collective memory of society.

How has history developed in health?

Historical approaches have been used for many decades in the study of health. The earliest studies celebrated the advances of medicine and saw the past in terms of historical progress to the present. Studies had titles like *The Romance of Medicine* or *Masters of Medicine*. This style of historical writing is known as *Whig history*, after the eighteenth-century British political party that presented a progressive view of British history.

Such history represented a view of the past that assumed that the present was right. It downplayed lay perspectives and those of non-medical workers. The history of medicine emerged as an academic discipline in the 1930s and 1940s. Early protagonists included Henry Sigerist who established the *Bulletin of the History of Medicine* at Johns Hopkins University in Baltimore in the United States in 1933; and George Rosen, whose *History of Public Health* (1958) was a major early book on the subject. Such historians argued that:

- doctors need critical awareness
- the past shapes the present
- medicine and science are not separate worlds but are enmeshed with society and politics.

The social history of medicine broadened the subject matter of history in health still further from the 1960s. It looked at population health and at demographic history, at health systems and the different health workers within them and at medical science, the 'framing of disease' and the role of innovation and application in medicine and health. Women and children in history and also lay perspectives on health were given historical attention. Social history used sociological and anthropological insights and theories. The aim was to place medicine and health within their political and social context.

Historical approaches

History is quite distinct from both the natural and other social sciences disciplines, although there are areas of overlap in terms of methods with the latter. Unlike the phenomena studied by natural scientists, all historical events are unique; history does not provide experiments that can be repeated. There are no predictive laws about human behaviour. Many historians argue that positivist claims have failed and that there can be no 'lessons' of history. This point is discussed below.

A key difference between history and some other social sciences is that historians do not generate data, and it is impossible in historical research to design an instrument that will elicit the dataset that you will require. Historians are always reliant on surviving sources. You cannot design a questionnaire to elicit standardized information. However, some research techniques are comparable; oral history interviews and 'witness seminars', for instance, have similarities to the in-depth interviews and focus groups used by social researchers. The purposes of these research methods, however, differ significantly from other social science usage, as discussed below.

The uses of history in health

History has been used in three main ways in the study of health.

The 'lesson of history'

This is the use of events in the past to support a present-day stance. Health history is often used in this way. Read the following claims about history:

- The struggles in nineteenth-century Britain by public health activists to secure clean water and sanitation in the new industrialized cities offer a 'lesson' for developing countries facing similar situations in the present.
- The history of liberal and non-punitive responses to venereal diseases in the nineteenth and early twentieth centuries in England provides a model for the developments of policies for HIV/AIDS.

✐ Activity 15.1

Think about this use of history as 'a lesson'. List its possible advantages and disadvantages to public health personnel.

↻ Feedback

Advantages could be:

• A clear model for action that has already been used and that worked.

Disadvantages could be:

- Over-simplification – there could be more than one 'lesson' from the past.
- The past should be looked at on its own terms and cannot easily be transferred to the present. Such an exercise is sometimes known as *'presentism'*.
- Historical models derived from Western countries may not be universally applicable in other contexts.

Journalist history: assigning blame in history

History is sometimes used to settle scores or to assign praise or blame. People use history, for instance, to argue that there was 'delay' in responding to certain health crises. The history of responses to tobacco is one example of this approach; and histories of HIV/AIDS have also argued that there was a delay in the early response. Such history again tends to be 'presentist' and to assume that our present-day perceptions also applied in the past. Some countries have used historical evidence as a means of feeding into current political realities in a different way. The Truth and Reconciliation Commission in South Africa is an example of this function; the evidence of people who took part in past events has been used as a way of healing differences and laying to rest the tensions of the past.

History to make you think

History can have a more challenging function, with an ability to counter current preconceptions. It can lead us to realize what our preconceptions are and how they have come about, and perhaps to question them. For example:

- Worboys (1988) has studied the rise of interest in colonial malnutrition in the interwar years. He has shown that this was not a matter of scientific progress, the uncovering of new scientific knowledge, but rather ideas arose out of the political realities of the day and in particular the relations between England and her colonies. The idea of malnutrition and its scientific definition established a particular way of looking at the issue. This stressed 'native ignorance' rather than structural issues.
- Berridge (1999) has analysed why drugs like opium and cocaine came to be restricted in the early twentieth century. She shows that the dangers of the drugs themselves were a secondary consideration and that other factors such as professional rivalries, class and race considerations and international power politics were more important in securing restriction.

Historical methods

Historians use two broad categories of data in order to analyse past events. *Primary sources* are the materials left by people who lived in the past. *Secondary sources* are the books and articles written by historians based on the primary sources.

When you begin to research or examine a public health issue or policy, you should first survey its *historiography*. Historiography is what historians have already written on the topic. This will give you an idea of what arguments have been made and what areas looked at. It establishes the framework for looking at the primary sources.

A range of primary sources can then be used. For the sake of clarity, three types are identified here:

- documentary
- quantitative
- oral.

In practice, historians often use a combination of different source material and rarely rely on one type of source alone.

Documentary sources

Documentary sources are a key resource for historical work. The following exercise will help you understand what this source can comprise.

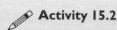 **Activity 15.2**

Look around the room you are sitting in or walk round your house or flat. Now imagine yourself in a health care setting such as a clinic, doctor's surgery or hospital. Or imagine you are sitting in the office of the minister of health of your country.

List some of the materials, the primary sources, which might be used by historians in 100 years' time to reconstruct and analyse what is happening now in these settings.

Feedback

In your home, there might be:

- an article on diet and health on a crisis in health services funding in a newspaper
- a packet of painkillers with instructions for taking them
- a TV programme about a health issue.

In the health setting, there might be:

- posters encouraging healthy eating
- your medical records (you cannot see these, except your own, but you know they are kept).

In the minister's office, there might be:

- a memo from the chief medical officer about the progress of an anti-malaria campaign
- a report on hospital reorganization from an independent research body.

This list could continue. The minister, for example, might write his/her autobiography after leaving office. What you have identified are all primary documentary sources.

There is a wide range of such sources:

- official sources such as state and local government reports and papers
- Newspapers, journals and literary sources
- letters and personal papers
- visual evidence such as art and also artefacts. Most historians concentrate on verbal documents using words, but the term can also be applied to visual materials as well.

Many historians use material collected in *archives*, which include:

- official government archives
- specialist archives (for example the archives of trade unions)
- local history archives
- newspaper archives.

Some of these archives will be generally open and accessible, whereas others may be more difficult to access. Material that contains patients' names is generally closed to public scrutiny and you have to seek permission for this.

Electronic documents are also now sources for historians. Television programmes are only partially archived and commercial companies may charge large fees to access their material. Material on the Internet is also accessed by historians and in recent years it has become possible to digitize documents so that they can be accessed online.

Quantitative sources

Some of the sources listed above may provide statistics about the past. There may be published statistics about causes of death and how these have changed over time. In Britain, the General Register Office was established in the 1830s thus long time series are available.

✏ Activity 15.3

What advantages and disadvantages are there in using data such as published statistics?

↻ Feedback

Advantages could be:

- The ability to discern long-term trends over time.
- A means of assessing contemporary perceptions against what was really happening.

Disadvantages could be:

- The issue of reliability. For example, cause of death data reflect the changing nature of disease classification over time and cannot be used without reference to that context.
- Assuming that quantitative sources offer greater certainty than other sources.

Statistical sources are also available within documentary material. For example, hospital yearbooks can be analysed to look at changes within the hospital over time. Records of lunatic asylums and mental hospitals have been analysed by historians to show the patterns of who was admitted to the asylum, how long they stayed and whether they were readmitted. This kind of statistical analysis, which is computer based, can contribute to discussions about the function of the asylum in the past and how it changed or was experienced differently by different sets of people.

A major approach within history using quantitative material is that of *historical demography*. Historians have used parish registers of births and deaths in order to assess the causes of population increase that fuelled the industrial revolution and the rise of cities in Britain in the nineteenth century. Such demographic work has concluded that population increase and industrialization in the late eighteenth and early nineteenth centuries in England was driven by a rise in fertility rather than by a decrease in mortality. Such conclusions have implications for those considering population increase in countries outside Britain today, although obviously the specific social, cultural and political contexts have to be taken into account when making comparisons.

Questioning the sources

Historians are especially aware of the need to look critically at their sources. Questions have to be asked that enable you to assess the significance and meaning of each source. You can ask the following questions about each of your documents:

- Who created or wrote this source?
- When and where did they write it?
- For whom was it intended?
- What was its purpose?
- What was its effect? (this of course is a bigger question)
- What does it tell you? (this may be the biggest question of all)

What you are trying to do is to understand the standpoint of the person who produced the document and how it sheds light on the issues in which you are interested. This does not mean that you should discard documents that show 'bias'. In the past, as now, everyone has a point of view and this may influence what is produced. You might think that more technical sources, for example data series or patient records, are 'unbiased' but they are not a full record of the truth either. We have discussed problems with data series and patient records do not tell us everything about a patient. They inevitably leave out more about the person than they include.

✏ Activity 15.4

Try this questioning exercise with any documentary source you have to hand. Potential sources could be a newspaper article, a programme you are watching on television, an organization's annual report or a health promotion leaflet.

Oral history

Much experience is neither quantified nor written down. Oral accounts can be revealing and usually these are gathered from individuals through interviewing. This limits current research to those who have been born within the last 90 years. However, there are also oral history archives in some countries where earlier interviews have been deposited and are available to researchers. There are different forms of oral history interviewing. We can identify three types:

- life history interviews
- key informant interviews
- witness seminars.

Life history interviews are an important use of oral history. The new social history of medicine tried to look at what was called 'history from below'. It wanted to reconstruct the experience of people who did not appear in the documentary sources. If you want to do this, you could interview lay people or patients about health experiences, or women practitioners and patients, who have been largely absent from the historical record. This use of history has spread widely and has been used by local history groups. It is also used in the care of the elderly in some countries; reminiscence professionals encourage elderly people to talk about their life histories as a means of maintaining mental alertness and interaction with others.

Key informant interviews. People may be interviewed because they have played a role in events, such as a scientific discovery, the establishment of a speciality, or key health policy decision making. The idea is not to explore the interviewees' whole life history but rather their involvement in a particular set of events.

Witness seminars are a relatively recent development within oral history. They are rather like a focus group in social science research. Participants are those who have been involved in a particular set of events; they discuss these events in a group discussion, which is then recorded and transcribed. The interaction between participants sometimes achieves more than might emerge from individual face-to-face interviews. Witness seminars for health topics have so far mainly dealt with events in countries in the West. For example one seminar has considered the changes in abortion law in Britain in the 1960s; another has looked at the 1979 Black Report on inequalities in health and the subsequent impact of the report on health research (Berridge and Blume 2003).

What makes a good oral history interview?

You need to decide who you are going to interview for the purposes of your research. If you are interested in the changing role of a professional group, then a quota sample using different categories over time might be appropriate. If your research is on health policy decision making, then there will be certain interviewees who must be approached; a sample survey will not do. Remember that arranging interviews, conducting the interview, possibly transcribing, or reading through your notes or listening to your tapes, are time consuming processes. So the numbers of interviews actually possible must be carefully considered.

You need to prepare ahead of the interview, deciding what issue to explore and what recording material to use. The compilation of notes during the interview is also a safety mechanism but takes skill. In all cases researchers should obtain consent from those they interview and guarantee anonymity where requested.

Ground rules for a good oral interview are similar to those in Chapter 6 on qualitative interviewing, such as the need to develop rapport with the interviewee and to adopt a non-judgemental and open-ended stance for questioning.

We have already discussed some of the limitations of oral history. You might now be able to think of others. Dependent on your time frame, you may be limited regarding who is available for interview; it is always best to interview the oldest first. Memory is selective and sometimes people imagine there was a 'golden age' in the past when things were better that they are now. In policy interviews, participants may use the interview to settle old scores, to present a view of events that they hope the researcher will use uncritically. Other interviewees may have become celebrities who have been interviewed too often. Such people often develop a standard official story, which they offer interviewers.

How to use sources

The discussion about documentary, qualitative and oral history sources makes it clear that all these sources must be used with care and their limitations appreciated at the outset. The historian's main task is the uncovering and examination of such evidence but this must then be compiled into a coherent analysis accessible to outside readers.

Historians do not start out with a hypothesis that they are testing. The approach is deductive through interaction with the source material. Evidence is always fragmentary, either because it has not survived, or because it has been selected in particular ways for deposit in an archive. Historians working on more recent history can find that they are overwhelmed by the amount of material and cannot possibly use it all. Historians must therefore be careful that they are weighing up different types of evidence and make sure they are not constructing an analysis that simply confirms their own preconceptions.

Historical truth is the existing consensus among historians based on corroboration from the sources.

Controversy and interpretation in history

There are thus many areas of controversy in history, in particular in health where such discussions often have implications for the present. Historians argue over interpretation for two main reasons:

* New sources, techniques or methodologies allow new questions to be asked and answered.
* Each particular generation will rewrite its history and different theories will influence the nature of the arguments made.

One particular example of this process is the historical debate about what is called the 'McKeown thesis'. Thomas McKeown (1976) argued that the decline in mortality visible during the late nineteenth century could not have been the result of health technologies or of public health interventions, but was the outcome of better nutrition and higher living standards at the end of the century. Simon Szreter (1988) has examined the classification of disease data in this period and has argued that certain diseases actually declined earlier than the official statistics would lead us to believe. Such reclassification leads to the conclusion that public health interventions did play a greater role and that better nutrition alone cannot be a sufficient explanation for mortality decline. This controversy in history has present-day implications. It could impact on international agencies and their donor strategies; it reintroduces the importance of state activity (as a major driver of environmental improvements, for instance) rather than placing stress only on the role of the market to drive improvements in public health.

So doing historical research is not just a question of 'uncovering the facts' as a kind of historical detective story. It involves discovering and examining evidence and then presenting that evidence in a coherent analytical form. History is both a body of knowledge and an area of disputed and changing interpretation. It is not simply the written record of the past, but an argument about the past, which can be relevant to the present.

Summary

All current health issues, policies and structures are based on the past and history has an important role to play in assessing current preconceptions. Historical work uses secondary and primary sources and the latter can be documentary, quantitative or oral. Historians use evidence as a means of constructing an interpretation of the past, and that interpretation is always open to challenge from fresh argument, which in its turn is evidence based.

References

Berridge V (1999) *Opium and the People. Opiate Use and Drug Control Policy in Nineteenth and Early Twentieth Century England*. Revised and expanded edition. London: Free Association Books.

Berridge V and Blume S (eds) (2003) *Poor Health. Social Inequality Before and After the Black Report*. London: Frank Cass.

McKeown T (1976) *The Modern Rise of Population*. London: Edward Arnold.

Szreter S (1988) The importance of social intervention in Britain's mortality decline, c. 1850–1914 : a re-interpretation of the role of public health. *Social History of Medicine* 1: 1–37.

Worboys M (1988) The discovery of colonial malnutrition between the wars, in Arnold D (ed) *Imperial Medicine and Indigenous Societies*. Manchester: Manchester University Press, pp. 208–25.

Further reading

James M (1994) Historical research methods, in McConway K (ed) *Studying Health and Disease*. Milton Keynes: Open University Press.

This is one of the few surveys of historical research methods for health.

Thompson P and Perks R (1993) *An Introduction to the Use of Oral History in the History of Medicine*. London: National Sound Archive.

An oral history introduction that concentrates on the 'life history' and 'history from below' uses of the method.

16 | Multi-method and multi-disciplinary approaches

Judith Green

Overview

This final chapter looks at approaches to studying health that draw on more than one method or discipline. In practice, research topics in public health often generate a series of questions that need more than one method to address them adequately. These methods may draw on techniques from a range of social science (and other) disciplines. Less commonly, research in public health also aims to integrate the perspectives of different disciplines. This chapter examines the benefits and challenges of different ways of combining methods and disciplinary approaches.

Learning objectives

After studying this chapter, you will be able to:

- appreciate the complementary role of different methods and disciplines in health research
- explain the possibilities and limitations of triangulation

Key terms

Multi-disciplinary Combining two or more different disciplines.

Triangulation Using different data sets, methods or approaches to improve the validity of findings.

When is it appropriate to use multiple methods?

Although this book has introduced some social science methods under the headings of 'qualitative' and 'quantitative' methods, it has also advocated combining methods when appropriate to improve our understanding of the complex web of factors that impact on health and health service use. The problems facing public health are increasingly complex, and many researchers have called for a range of methodological strategies to be used to address them adequately (see, for example, Baum 1995). Identifying needs for interventions might typically require qualitative work alongside epidemiological surveys, and then a mixed method approach to evaluating the intervention, in for instance using epidemiological methods to measure outcomes (such as disease incidence) and qualitative methods to explore process and users' views of the intervention.

In such situations it is relatively unproblematic to see that different research designs and methods of data collection might need to be used within one project, or a series of projects. Public health professionals utilize research from a range of different perspectives in planning and delivering health care: from basic medical sciences, epidemiology, and economics as well as the social science disciplines that have been introduced in this book. Increasingly, we need skills in both understanding research findings from diverse perspectives, and thinking broadly about the most appropriate combinations of methods to use in any one project. In practice, many public health research programmes involve the use of a range of disciplines or methods working together, and most projects will draw on research findings from other disciplines. If we begin by thinking broadly about the combination of qualitative and quantitative methodological strategies within research programmes, there are perhaps a number of logical combinations, including:

- Using qualitative data *to inform* quantitative studies. For instance, when developing a quality-of-life outcome instrument, or a survey questionnaire, it is necessary to undertake detailed qualitative work to identify the main domains that are salient for the target group, and to explore the kind of language they use to describe them.
- Using qualitative work *to add depth* to statistics, or to explore why variables are related. In Chapter 5, an ethnographic investigation into sudden infant death syndrome was summarized. This used qualitative methods to examine epidemiological findings.
- Using quantitative work (such as a survey) to test the *generalizability* of small-scale qualitative studies.
- Using qualitative and quantitative work in tandem *to help validate* findings. Here, the strengths of one design or data collection method are used to offset the weaknesses of another. In Chapter 12, for instance, we mentioned a study by Campbell and Stone on how they used ethnographic methods to estimate the non-sampling error in survey work in Nepal. Here two different methods of finding out about knowledge of family planning (ethnographic fieldwork and surveys) were used.

Improving validity through triangulation

One common justification for using different data sets, methods or approaches within a study is to increase the validity of the findings, or our confidence in their credibility. This is called *triangulation*. Triangulation is built on the assumption that using two different 'readings' of one phenomenon will improve accuracy. An example of the use of different designs in tandem for increasing validity comes from Brent Wolff and colleagues (Wolff *et al.* 1993), who were interested in the relationship between family size and socioeconomic wellbeing in rural Thailand. Specifically, they wanted to explore the relationship between completed family size and outcomes such as the educational attainment of children, material wealth of the household and women's economic activity. They decided to run focus groups and a survey concurrently in order to generate two sets of data on the same phenomena. The focus groups enabled the researchers to explore perceptions of family size and wellbeing, whereas the survey aimed to gather objective measures of family composition and economic activity. In order to enhance the comparability of the findings from the two data sets, the researchers chose focus group participants from the survey respondents. There are a number of ways, claim Wolff and colleagues, that the two sets of data can be used to strengthen the credibility of the findings of the research overall. First, where focus group findings and survey findings confirm each other, we can have increased faith that we have valid data. One example the researchers in this case gave was data on who paid for children's education. Both survey results and focus group discussions suggested that this was exclusively the responsibility of the parents. Second, the focus group discussions help validate the survey when they provide contextual data to explain apparent anomalies. Third, the survey can provide detailed data on individual birth and work histories that allow statistical analysis, which could not be provided by focus groups. Using qualitative approaches thus strengthens our faith in the contextual detail provided, whereas the quantitative approach strengthens representativeness, and offsets the limits to generalizability typical in small scale qualitative studies. As Wolff *et al.* conclude:

> When they are concurrently designed and implemented, focus groups and surveys provide asymmetrical but independent observations of the study population that strengthen the ability to draw conclusions as well as confidence in the conclusions themselves. When surveys and focus groups point to the same conclusions, the results of independent analyses tend to confirm each other. When analysis of either one appears to be internally inconsistent or contradictory, the other source of data may help to elaborate or clarify the underlying mechanisms that produce these inconsistencies. (1993: 133)

Communicating across disciplines

Different research designs or data-collection methods can, then, complement each other in the same study, or be used in sequence to build up our knowledge of public health. Although it might appear to be straightforward to use different designs or disciplines in one project when they are each contributing to answering one particular question, in practice it can be very difficult to work in multi-disciplinary teams, or even to communicate findings effectively across disciplines.

✎ Activity 16.1

What barriers do you think there might be to effective multi-disciplinary working in health research?

↻ Feedback

Those trained in one discipline may find it difficult to present their work in ways that those from another discipline will understand. Some methodological starting points may be incompatible, such as a strong relativist and a positivist position. Additionally, some research designs are more widely accepted by policy makers and funders than others, and qualitative social scientists may find it more difficult to obtain funding for their research. Chapter 2 introduced some of these epistemological differences: these can be real barriers to multi-disciplinary work, and most researchers find that building up trust and mutual understanding takes considerable time and resources.

A first challenge is communication. Public health researchers are often skilled at disseminating findings to those within their own discipline but may be less skilled at presenting findings to those who are unused to the particular vocabularies, theoretical models or favoured data-collection methods of that discipline. The following is an example of a project that was both multi-method and multi-disciplinary in which the anthropologists Scrimshaw and Hurtado (1988) had to consider how to disseminate their findings in appropriate ways to those from other disciplines.

Presenting anthropological findings to project planners

The Central American Diarrheal Disease Control Project, described by Susan Scrimshaw and Elena Hurtado, involved a number of different disciplines and research methods, including basic research on pathogens that caused diarrhoeal disease, development of effective rehydration therapies and monitoring of child health in the area as well as anthropological research on folk health beliefs. Scrimshaw and Hurtado argue that, to be useful, the findings of anthropologists need to be presented in ways that health care planners and providers can use. In their study, they note a detailed knowledge of local health beliefs, culture and language for effective health interventions – in this case the introduction of oral rehydration therapy (ORT) to treat diarrhoeal disease. Although it is vital to know local terms for different kinds of diarrhoea in order to target health promotion effectively, and to understand local health beliefs about both the causes and potential cures, the kind of anthropological research that produces this knowledge may not be accessible for health planners not familiar with anthropological writing. As a contribution to a programme on reducing the morbidity from diarrhoeal disease in Central America, the research team collated information on 'ethnoclassifications', or folk taxonomies, of diarrhoea in communities in Guatemala and Costa Rica. These proved to be complex. One classification, from a highland community in Guatemala, identified eight different kinds of diarrhoea, distinguished by their primary cause: the mother, food, tooth eruption, fallen fontanel or stomach, evil eye, stomach worms, cold or dysentery. These primary classifications were further subdivided, and different therapies were deemed appropriate for different causes. One example was diarrhoea caused by the mother being 'overheated' (from pregnancy or being out on a hot day), which might spoil her milk. In this case, the folk remedy would be to abstain from breastfeeding, or to wean the baby. The only type of diarrhoea that was seen as appropriate to take to the clinic was that of dysentery, which was the most serious form and distinguished by blood in the stools. Others were seen as amenable to home cures (such as herbal teas, baths and massages) and various traditional healers.

These kinds of findings have significant implications for project planners. To be effective, health promotion has to reflect the different kinds of diarrhoea in the local folk classifications and terminology, and make it clear that rehydration is still needed for forms of diarrhoea that are seen as less serious than dysentery. Scrimshaw and Hurtado (1988) stress the need to present anthropological findings in ways that workers from other disciplines can understand. There were a number of strategies that aided the utilization of ethnographic findings in this project. First, the researchers trained fieldworkers to carry out similar projects to map the folk taxonomies of the communities they worked with, and in one area clinic workers were trained to carry out rapid assessment of community beliefs. A newsletter to the wider project team regularly carries findings from the ethnographic projects. Joint workshops with clinicians and health educators were used to look at ways of integrating the findings. Rather than expecting project staff from other disciplines to read lengthy anthropological monographs, the researchers summarized the ethnoclassifications briefly as taxonomies, with diagrams if possible. These were presented at meetings wherever possible, with time to discuss them.

Activity 16.2

1   How did anthropological fieldwork inform the disease control project?
2   What factors do the authors think contributed to their influence on other professionals involved with this project?

Feedback

1 Anthropologists found that the way in which people classified diarrhoeal diseases was more complex than planners predicted, and only some causes were seen as reason to visit the primary health care post. Lay beliefs exist outside the formal sector, however well educated a population is. Their findings have informed the delivery of care and influenced the form of a survey; they have also had an impact on training in the countries within the project.

2 The authors attribute their relative success in this multi-disciplinary setting to several factors:

  • meetings and workshops that included those from other disciplines
  • the researchers' willingness to present findings in a clear and useful way.

In the case study you have just read, the key issue of combining the findings from ethnographic research into a broader project was that of *presenting* the research in ways that those trained in other disciplines could understand easily so that they could integrate the implications into their own work. In other multi-disciplinary studies, the differences between traditions may be more fundamental, and concern the epistemological underpinnings of different designs, as was discussed in Chapter 2. This has both advantages and a challenge for social scientists working in public health. The advantages are, first, that these differences can be used to help validate, or strengthen the credibility of findings through triangulation, as discussed above. Second, we can increase the complexity of our explanations, by using different designs to address different aspects of the question. The challenges though, relate to the difficulties of doing this in practice. We cannot assume that data sets generated from different designs will confirm each other in any simplistic way, and often a more complex understanding of the meaning of different sets of findings from different studies is needed.

The limits to triangulation

As the example of Brent Wolff and colleagues (1993) research in Thailand, summarized earlier, suggests, multiple methods within one study are often advocated as a way of *triangulating* results. If the different methods produce similar results, our confidence in those results can be greater. If they don't, and we have greater faith in the validity of one method (as Campbell and Stone did in their study in Nepal), one method can be used to estimate the limitations of the other.

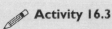 **Activity 16.3**

Birthweight is widely used as an outcome measure in health research. If you were using published statistics on birthweight to look at health care needs within a geographical area, how might you use other methods to validate the weights recorded?

 Feedback

Some possibilities are:

- using participant observation in maternity wards to explore how reliably birth weight is recorded by ward staff
- interviewing administrators responsible for recording birth data to find out how the demands of their job influence the recording of birth weight.

One example of a study that used qualitative methods to validate health data comes from Gillian Lewando-Hundt and colleagues (1999). They were interested in mother and child health in Gaza, where the political and social context influenced administrative records in a number of ways. First, the researchers noted that when they looked at addresses on the register of births, none were complete. The research team found that most street names and numbers in the Gaza Strip were removed during the Intifada, and few were replaced at the time of the fieldwork. There were also economic disincentives to providing an address in the Gaza Strip, as employees who live outside the area receive a transport allowance for travelling to work in the city. Furthermore, the Ministry of Interior regulations state that birth certificates are only valid if the baby has the same address as the father, so if the father has moved (and this is a highly mobile population) the address given on the birth certificate is likely to be wrong, as hospital clerks merely recorded them from the father's (often out-of-date) identity card. The research team also looked at birth weight records. They found that hospital discharge forms often missed out this piece of information, so the clerk responsible for completing records would just type '3 kg' if the data were missing. As Lewando-Hundt and colleagues note, the official statistics might then seriously underestimate the rate of low birth weight in this area. Thus detailed qualitative work allowed the research team to see what limitations there might be in the official statistics, and to identify some ways of improving record keeping. They conclude:

> Qualitative research has a role to play in contextualising the process and meaning of vital registration at a local and national level . . . we need to coordinate the bureaucratic and the familial levels so that statistics will be more culturally valid, accurate and humane . . .
>
> Anthropology can make its contribution to epidemiology. It is precisely here that qualitative research can be used to validate health surveillance data and guide policy interventions.

In this example, different sources of data, such as observations of the actual work of recording statistics, were used to understand the process better, and therefore the validity of health data. The logic of this approach is that the strengths of one method help counterbalance the weaknesses of another. Thus, interviews with patients can be used to collect the detailed data on health care experiences that might be missing from hospital records, or observations used on a few hospital wards to validate the replies of hospital managers in a national survey.

Activity 16.4

Consider the following scenario: a student interested in the prevalence of health behaviours that prevent diarrhoeal illness interviewed a sample of 30 mothers. Most of them understood the risks of diarrhoea and how to prevent it. They claimed to wash their hands before preparing food, after changing babies' nappies and after using the lavatory. She validated these results by observing mothers at social functions and in their homes, but found that in practice few mothers washed their hands. Can you think of any problems with methodological triangulation of this sort?

Feedback

It is difficult to judge between the different findings that may be generated by different methods. Although the student was using two methods to answer the same question, interviews are not really an appropriate method for gaining data on behaviour. Instead, these data are really about 'beliefs': what, for instance, the mothers believe to be good practice.

What this example points to is the 'contextual' nature of human action. What we say and do are situated in specific social contexts. Although triangulation can provide useful additional data, problems can be encountered when using it in any simplistic way to validate accounts. Different methods address different questions, so it is not surprising that the answers are different. However, using multiple methods is a good way to add depth to research, and to investigate more facets of the same problem.

Different methods, different data

As an example of how different methods produce different data, consider Hilary Graham's (1987) study of why some low-income women in Britain continue to smoke. This is an example of qualitative research being used to unpack the findings of quantitative studies (that smoking in women in the UK is associated with low income), and of the use of multiple methods in one study. She used:

- diaries, which women completed over 24 hours to collect data on their daily routines
- the Nottingham Health Profile (NHP), a self-administered questionnaire designed to measure subjective health status
- in depth interviews.

All these methods have their limitations: interviews, for instance, however carefully conducted, can only provide a snapshot of everyday life. However, these different methods cannot 'validate' each other in any simplistic way, as they address different aspects of Graham's research question. The NHP can provide quantitative data on how women perceive their own health, and could be used to compare the self-rated health of smokers and non-smokers in the sample, and those on low and higher incomes. The interviews and diaries could be used to provide detailed data on the everyday experiences of women, and there were some interesting differences in the data the two methods provided. Graham reports: 'Compared to statements made in interviews about smoking behaviour, there was a significant under-reporting of smoking in the diaries of those who smoked. Unless smoking was reported as the "main" activity, it tended not to be reported' (1987: 52).

However, this does not invalidate the data from diaries. It provides Graham with a clue to the meaning of her data. She notes that smoking is intricately tied to the routines of everyday life: the cigarettes that are 'noticed' and therefore recorded in the diary are those that mark the breaks in the routines of housework and child care. Data from the interviews provided detailed accounts of how women coped in poverty, and the meaning of smoking in their lives. Thus, the interview data did not 'invalidate' the diaries: it provided data on a rather different aspect of the research question and enabled Graham to explore the data in more depth.

Triangulation is thus not a simple process of building up multiple accounts of one phenomenon from different perspectives in the hope that they somehow 'match' and that we can therefore have more faith in the results. Rather, it is a more subtle process through which researchers can explore the differences, and build up a more complex picture of health or health behaviour.

Summary

Health behaviour is complex and is influenced by many factors. Using different research designs and data-collection methods, and drawing on the perspectives of different disciplines can add to our understanding of the relationships between these influences. Key issues for multi-method and multi-disciplinary projects are finding ways to integrate not only the findings but also the theoretical perspectives of different approaches.

References

Baum F (1995) Researching public health: behind the qualitative-quantitative methodological debate. *Social Science and Medicine* 40: 459–68.

Graham H (1987) Women's smoking and family health. *Social Science and Medicine* 25: 47–56.

Lewando-Hundt G, Abed Y, Skeik M, Beckerleg S and El Alem A (1999) Addressing birth in Gaza: using qualitative methods to improve vital registration. *Social Science and Medicine* 48: 833–43.

Scrimshaw S and Hurtado E (1988) Anthropological involvement in the central American diarrhoeal disease control project. *Social Science and Medicine* 27: 97–105.

Wolff B, Knodel J, Sittitari W (1993) Focus groups and surveys as complementary research methods. In Morgan DL (ed) *Successful Focus Groups: Advancing the State of the Art.* Newbury Park, CA: Sage.

Further reading

Bryman A (1988) *Quality and Quantity in Social Research.* London: Unwin Hyman.

This is a more theoretical discussion of qualitative and quantitative paradigms in the social sciences.

Janes CR, Stall R and Gifford S (1986) *Anthropology and Epidemiology: Interdisciplinary Approaches to the Study of Health and Disease.* Dordrecht: D. Reidel Publishing Company

This has some interesting case studies of how anthropology can be integrated with epidemiology, and some material on the history of collaboration between the disciplines.

Glossary

Archive A formal location where documentary and visual materials are gathered together and organized. It may also refer to a private individual's collection of personal papers, or to an electronic archive, where materials on a topic are available online.

Closed question Question on a questionnaire or interview schedule that gives the respondent a predetermined choice of responses.

Coding In qualitative analysis, the process by which data extracts are labelled as indicators of a concept.

Concepts The phenomena that the researcher is interested in (such as 'inequalities in health' or 'social status'), which are not directly observable but which are assumed to exist because they give rise to measurable phenomena.

Controlled experiment A research design in which outcomes in the experimental group are compared to those in a 'control' group.

Deliberative methods Those that enable the participants to develop their own views as part of the process.

Documentary sources All sources of information that are written or printed. They may be verbal or visual.

Explanatory model Systematic set of knowledge, beliefs and attitudes with regard to a particular illness which offers explanations of illness and treatment to guide choices among available therapies and to cast personal and social meaning on the experience of illness.

Focus groups Groups of people brought together to discuss a topic, with one or more facilitators who introduce and guide the discussion and record it in some way.

Generalizability In survey research, the extent to which the results from a sample survey can be applied to the whole population.

Historical demography The construction and use of historical data sets to examine issues of mortality, morbidity and fertility.

Historiography The study of what secondary sources say about an historical subject and how this interpretation has changed.

Hypothesis A provisional explanation for the phenomenon being studied.

Illness behaviour The way a person behaves when they feel a need for better health.

In-depth interviews The interviewer uses a topic list, but respondents' priorities influence the final range of questions covered.

Indicators The empirical attributes of variables that can be observed and measured (such as 'blood pressure' or 'monthly wage').

Interaction Communication between people.

Interpretative approaches Approaches that focus on understanding human behaviour from the perspective of those being studied.

Measurement scale The level of measurement used (nominal, ordinal, ratio, interval).

Medical pluralism The existence of more than one medical tradition. Nearly all societies are medically pluralistic.

Medical systems Sets of premises and ideas that enable people to organize their perceptions and experiences of medical events (for example illness episodes) and to organize their interventions for affecting and controlling these events.

Medical traditions Distinctive combination of ideas, practices, skills, tools and materials that are related to recognizing, explaining and treating illness conditions.

Medical sectors Components that make up the medical system, usually including a *popular* sector (lay, non-professional), a *folk* sector (non-professional, specialist) and *professional* sectors (organized, institutionalized).

Method A set of strategies for asking useful questions, designing a study, collecting data and analysing data.

Methodology The study of the principles of investigation, including the philosophical foundations of choice of methods.

Multi-disciplinary Combining two or more different disciplines.

Natural groups Groups which occur 'naturally', such as workmates or household members.

Naturalism Studying social behaviour in the context in which it 'naturally' occurs.

Non-sampling error The amount of error in the data we have collected that is due to problems with the reliability and validity of our data collection instrument (as opposed to problems with our sampling of the population).

Open question A question on a questionnaire or interview schedule that allows the respondent to give any answer.

Operationalizing The process of identifying the appropriate variables from concepts or constructs and finding adequate and specific indicators of variables.

Oral history Interview-based recollection of events in the past.

Patterns of resort The paths people make as they pick and choose their ways from one sector of the medical system to another, in search of diagnosis, treatment and other services.

Positivism A philosophy of science that assumes that reality is stable and can be researched by measuring observable indicators.

Presentism A view of historical events that takes its reference point from the present-day situation, rather than trying to assess the past on its own terms.

Primary historical sources The materials that historians find and use in their research. These are the evidence on which historians base their arguments.

Probability sample Each member of the population has a random and equal chance of being selected.

Qualitative Pertaining to the nature of phenomena: how they are classified.

Quantitative Pertaining to the measurement of phenomena.

Rapport Relaxed, natural communication between interviewer and respondent.

Reliability The extent to which an instrument produces consistent results.

Response rate The proportion of those sampled who responded.

Sample Group of respondents drawn from a population to represent the whole.

Sampling error Limitations on how far inferences from a sample can be generalized to the whole population.

Secondary historical sources In historical research, what other historians have written about the past.

Semi-structured interviews The interviewer uses a guide in which set questions are covered, but can prompt for more information.

Structured interviews The interviewer uses a schedule in which questions are read out in a predetermined order.

Therapy management group The set of individuals involved in diagnosing the cause and consequence of affliction, making choices about the therapeutic options to adopt and directing the course of therapy.

Triangulation Using different data sets, methods or approaches to improve the validity of findings.

Validity The extent to which an indicator measures what it intends to measure.

Variables Aspects of phenomena that change (such as 'disease severity' or 'income').

Whig history A view of history that assumes the past is a process of inevitable progress to the present.

Index

Page numbers in *italics* refer to tables, and activity and feedback boxes.